AF711928

How To Stop Poising Yourself

The Pure & Natural Way

A Guide To Avoiding
Processed, Commercialized,
Irradiated, & Genetically
Engineered Food and Products

Compiled by
Nasir Makr Hakim
&
Rose Hakim

Published by
Secretarius MEMPS Publications
5025 N Central Ave #415 • Phoenix, AZ 85012
Phone & Fax (602) 466-7347
Email: cs@memps.com
www.memps.com

Copyright © 2008
Secretarius MEMPS Publications

All rights reserved.
No part of this book may be reproduced
in any form, except for the
inclusion of brief quotations in
reviews, without permission
in writing from the author/publisher.

ISBN 13 978-1-884855-99-3
ISBN 10 1-884855-99-7

PRINTED IN THE UNITED STATES OF AMERICA

Table of Contents

Introduction

Messenger Elijah Muhammad's books, How To Eat To Live, Books 1 & 2, were first published in 1967 and 1972 respectively and Jethro Kloss's book, Back To Eden followed soon thereafter. These were just a few of the various books on the market instructing us on how to eat and prepare our meals. As well, Elijah Muhammad's books not only pointed out good foods and means of preparation, but he went a few steps further with warnings about the process and commercialization of future foods to come. In this book, We make no attempt at reinterpreting, reinventing or improving upon what he or Kloss wrote. The objective of this book is only to make the reader aware of the means and ways the food and their by-products have been adversely transformed since the time of their initial publications. From this awareness and updated information contained herein, it will enable the reader to stay consistent with the good and correct principles taught in those writings.

We felt there was a great need for a writing such as this, because through processing and commercialization, food has taken on a different form from what we had grown accustomed to.

Since the 60's and 70's, foods that were once called "pure" and "natural" no longer qualify for this definition. Various government agencies responsible for checking the safety of food have adopted various definitions for political and economic reasons, but at the expense of our health. Consequently, the word pure simply means that there are "acceptable" levels of toxins, or acceptable levels of mercury, or acceptable levels of pesticides, herbicides or solvents per part, per million.

There was a time when brown sugar was a lot healthier than sugar is today. What was once stated as brown sugar was simply "raw sugar." It was a lot healthier and when Elijah Muhammad, for example, recommended it, he did not mean what today has come to be known as brown sugar, which is highly refined white sugar with molasses poured over it. For on one hand he would not advise us to NOT eat refined products while simultaneously telling us to eat the new form of brown sugar.

As well, take for instance the aspect of pork. Many religious people as well as commoners who do not eat meat are not aware that many of the foods they consume on a daily basis are filled with meat and pork by-products. For Muslims, Jews and other religious folks, this so-called food (pork) is completely prohibited due to God's forbidding and the indestructible worm inside. It is to never be taken for food, so much so, Elijah Muhammad advises that his followers should die first before eating it.

In today's market, there are hundreds of thousands of products that are made from pork and its by-products. Since the 60's, these products are not so well pointed out. These are just a few of the reasons this book is essential and will serve as an excellent source of food safety information.

There are two main veins this book will pursue: one is the processes used to manufacture, store and preserve food and the surrounding equipment associated and secondly, the commercialization of it for maximum profits at the expense of the people's health in general. Of course, secondary to this is the fact that bad food equals bad health, which equals a great economic boom in medicine, doctors and hospitalization. Not only will this book enlightened the reader as to the problems, but it will also furnish solutions in the form of alternatives.

We trust the reader will find great benefit in this book.

HOW TO USE THIS BOOK

This book would be considerably more beneficial if used as a reference book. Additionally, it will serve to make you aware of current misunderstanding and misconceptions about food, cosmetics, equipment and the terms surrounding them.

It will serve to orientate the novice who wants to start practicing better health. For those already practicing the principles of good health and diet, it will update your current knowledge base with newly researched information about various elements and aspects rarely found in other books. The long-term practitioner will find the means to enhance their experience and include very important data to their research for continued personal development and general education. Lastly, there is online links, which have many of the items cited in this book available along with their sources.

The basis of eating should be as a way of life and not a diet. For thousands of years mankind has been searching for the key to life or the fountain of youth; as well, in religious circles, the promise of a better life is expected. Yet, few understood it to come from simply knowing how to eat to live. This is from where the abundance of life promised in the scriptures would come.

The knowledge of how to eat and what to eat has been kept back and hidden from the people for thousands of years. The sick have been held hostage for their money or intangible assets since time immemorial. Doctors, even primitive and natural healers, surround themselves with mystery as they use herbs or chemicals and incantations or “prognoses” to help the sick recover.

This guide is designed to aid you in understanding that if you cannot grow your own food or make your own external health care products, then knowing where and how to identify and acquire the best on the market with minimal cost will be the next best option. Bear in mind that food has been degraded by modern processes and is no longer considered “pure” or “natural” anymore. The objective of this book is to assist you in getting the best food available. Lastly, when we say minimal cost, we mean that either you will pay premium cost for the best food today to stay healthy as possible, or you will pay outrageous prices at the hands of doctors, surgeons and the pharmaceutical companies.

We deliberately choose not to mention specific philosophies, people and organizations behind the intentional concealing of knowledge of what and how to eat to live.

LITTLE PURE FOOD ON THE MARKET

God's Messengers and Prophets have universally pointed to us that there is no way we can ever enjoy good health unless we obey the teacher of health. They teach that God knows the histories of how people practiced their way of life for as far back into the hundreds of thousands, millions and billions of years. Should He not know the best way to eat to live?

Since coming from the country sides into the concrete cities for factory work, finding ways produce large quantities in as little time as possible has been the driving force behind food producers. Making food have more shelf life for the purpose of preservation and extended travel has culminated into a vast array of experimentation. They are experimenting on your life to see what will take you away and what will keep you here for a certain length of time. Our lives have become dependent and limited by the food we eat that is prepared by people who are racing with time.

Limited time and limited knowledge has forced them to experiment on themselves and us too. It is true that the earth provides the healthiest food possible for human consumption; however, with the advent of the age of industrialization came a move away from proper dieting and food preparation, to an explosion of processes to make food easier and quicker to prepare and eat. Consequently "fast food" produced in the least time as possible has been accomplished but at the price of good health. Every day it seems there is a new commercial with different acronyms for diseases never heard of before. Is it that these new diseases came from another planet or simple have fallen from the sky? No, most are due to the new type of "so-called food" on the market, the processes used to mass-produce it and the measures adopted to maintain and preserve it for long shelf life.

The very earth is now poisoned from experimentation on the food grown for the markets, because it is the almighty dollar or commercialization sought and not almighty health and long life for you and me.

Although the food that comes from the earth is natural, it is poisoned in other ways and through various processes. Additives, chemicals, irradiation, pesticides, pollution, and residue from solvents and various parasites are all poisonous.

Personal experience with eating, coupled with deliberate and constant awareness of food manufacturing, preparation and processing, has brought about startling discoveries. Not only has food been degraded to the extent of not even being food anymore, foods labeled as "pure" and "natural" have become as poisonous if not more poisoned the what's deemed "regular."

This book addresses the need to keep up with and versed in the new means and methods "food" is being dumped into the human food chain. Pursuing up to date knowledge about the deceptive practices surrounding food and the mislabeling, have become paramount in our quest to keep up with modern times and techniques.

Healthy alternatives for obsolete products, updated information for altered products and comprehensive information regarding modern poisons have been furnished in this book for the reader's safety.

FOOD ADDITIVES

We often think of food additives as complex chemical substances produced by our modern society. However, the use of food additives dates back to ancient times. Early people used salt to preserve meat and fish, herbs and spices to season foods, sugar to preserve fruits, and vinegar to pickle cucumbers.

Today American food manufacturers use nearly 3000 direct food additives. Some of these additives sound familiar like salt, sugar, yeast and vanilla. Others have complex scientific names that may sound unfamiliar, like ascorbic acid, butylated hydroxyanisol (BHA), sodium benzoate, sodium erythorbate and carageenan. Whether familiar or not, all food additives serve a useful function and must be approved by the Food and Drug Administration (FDA) before they can be included in food.

What Are Food Additives?

A food additive is any substance that becomes part of a food product either directly or indirectly during some phase of processing, storing or packaging. Additives can either be derived from naturally occurring or synthetic materials. Direct additives are purposefully added to food in very small quantities as a result of growing, processing or packaging

Food additives can only be used for specific purposes. They must serve a useful function. Manufacturers cannot use additives to deceive the consumer by disguising faulty processing or concealing damage or spoilage, nor if alternative manufacturing practices are available that are both safe and economical. Nor can food additives be used if they significantly decrease the nutritional value of the food.

Why Are Food Additives Used?

Food additives perform a number of functions in food. In general, they can be divided into five categories:

- Preservatives help to keep food fresh and prevent spoilage by controlling bacteria, mold, fungi, yeast or chemical changes.
- Nutrients maintain or improve the nutritional quality of food. For example, vitamins and minerals are added to many common foods like milk, flour, cereal and margarine to make up for those likely to be lacking in a person's diet or lost in food processing.
- Processing aids make products more pleasing by improving the consistency, providing body, adding stability, helping oil and water mix, retaining moisture, or preventing lumping.
- Flavors complement, magnify or modify the taste and aroma of a food. These can include spices, flavor enhancers, natural and synthetic flavors and sweeteners.
- Colors give foods a desired, appetizing or characteristic color.

Using food additives enables manufacturers to produce and distribute convenience foods with increased shelf life and decreased waste. Stabilizers and preservatives make it possible to ship a wide variety of foods all over the world.

The FDA determines, based on the best scientific data available, if the additive is safe under the proposed conditions of use. If the FDA approves an additive, it issues regulations that may include: the type of food the additive can be used in; the maximum amounts to be used; and the labeling requirements.

The United States Department of Agriculture (USDA) must also authorize additives that are proposed for use in meat and poultry products. After approving a new additive, government officials monitor consumption and keep track of any new research on its safety. The FDA also operates an Adverse Reaction Monitoring System (ARMS) to investigate complaints from consumers, physicians or food companies regarding food additives. The ARMS database helps officials track complaints and determine if a reported adverse reaction represents a real public health hazard associated with food.

There are two categories of food additives that are not subject to the testing and approval process, "prior sanctioned" and “GRAS” substances. Substances designated as "prior sanctioned" were approved by the FDA before the 1958 Food Additives Amendment. GRAS additives (Generally Recognized As Safe) have been extensively used in the past with no known harmful effect and are believed to be safe. Substances on the GRAS list have been under review since 1969 to ensure their safety. Yet, it is under this umbrella most abuses have and are taking place.

Under the guise of this government agency, the entire food chain is at the mercy of corporations and their practices of commercialization.

Melamine

Uses

Melamine is used combined with formaldehyde to produce melamine resin, a very durable thermosetting plastic, and of melamine foam, a polymeric cleaning product. The end products include countertops, fabrics, glues and flame retardants. Melamine is one of the major components in Pigment Yellow 150, a colorant in inks and plastics.

Melamine is also used to make fertilizers.

Melamine derivatives of arsenical drugs are potentially important in the treatment of African trypanosomiasis.

Toxicity

Little is known with respect to melamine toxicity in human subjects. Animal studies have shown that melamine is not metabolized in rats, and is excreted unchanged.

Acute (brief or severe) Toxicity

Melamine is reported to have an oral LD50 of >3000 mg/kg based on rat data, which makes it only minimally toxic or as "minimally toxic" as table salt, which has a similar LD50 value. It is also an irritant when inhaled or in contact with the skin or eyes. The reported dermal LD50 is >1000mg/kg for rabbits. In a 1945 study, large doses of melamine were given orally to rats, rabbits and dogs with "no significant toxic effects" observed.

Chronic (having long duration) Toxicity

Ingestion of melamine may lead to reproductive damage, or bladder or kidney stones, which can lead to bladder cancer.

Official US statements

On April 27 US FDA subjected all vegetable proteins imported from China, intended for human or animal consumption, to detention without physical examination, including: Wheat Gluten, Rice Gluten, Rice Protein, Rice Protein Concentrate, Corn Gluten, Corn Gluten Meal, Corn By-Products, Soy Protein, Soy Gluten, Proteins (includes amino acids and protein hydrosylates), and Mung Bean Protein.

On April 28, the U.S. Department of Agriculture (USDA) and the FDA, in a joint press release acknowledged that pork from hogs fed melamine-contaminated feed had entered the human food supply, stating: "Based on information currently available, FDA and USDA believe the likelihood of illness after eating pork from swine fed the contaminated product would be very low."

On April 30, the USDA and the FDA updated their April 28 food safety position to include poultry, reflecting contaminated feed being fed to chickens in Indiana.

On May 7, the USDA and the FDA issued a joint press release reflecting the combined judgment of five federal agencies with regard to the risk to humans in consuming meat from animals fed feed contaminated with tainted pet food scraps, concluding: "There is very low risk to human health" in such cases involving pork and poultry. The risk assessment was conducted by scientists from FDA, the Food Safety and Inspection Service (FSIS) of USDA, CDC, the Environmental Protection Agency (EPA), and U.S. Customs and Border Protection: "In the most extreme risk assessment scenario, when scientists assumed that all the solid food a person consumes in an entire day was contaminated with melamine at the levels observed in animals fed contaminated feed, the potential exposure was about 2,500 times lower than the dose considered safe" using criteria established prior to current research focusing on the apparent increased toxicity related to the interaction of melamine and cyanuric acid in vivo, for which there is no established safe dosage. FDA and USDA are in the process of identifying a group of experts to convene a scientific advisory board that would be charged with reviewing the risk assessment and contributing to future scientific analysis related to the risk of melamine and its compounds to humans and animals.

Risks to human health from this mode of entering the human food supply have been said to be low according to a number of FDA, CDC and university toxicologists, though it was acknowledged that how melamine had harmed cats and dogs remains something of a mystery.

On May 10, on further inquiry into the risk to animal and human health of ingesting melamine and cyanuric acid in combination, Dr. David Acheson, Assistant Commissioner for Food Protection with the FDA said: "I'm not aware of any published studies on that. I have seen some preliminary data that would indicate that they are additive. When you put the two together, they are additive rather than synergistic.... The risk assessors also estimated that even if synergism were to occur, it would be unlikely to result in more than a tenfold increase in overall toxicity, and that still gives you a very large margin of safety." No data supporting additivity was produced at this time. No basis for estimating a tenfold increase in risk in the case of synergism was offered.

On May 15 USDA announced that pigs that ate melamine-tainted food has been cleared for human consumption. About 56,000 pigs have been affected in several states. However, no tests have been carried out on the effects of cyanuric acid in pork as well as possible affects of interaction with melamine in the body. While the statement also said that there is no evidence of bioaccumulation of melamine alone, no mention was made whether bioaccumulation might be affected by the interaction of melamine and cyanuric acid in vivo.

In addition to now testing a wide variety of imported food products and ingredients for melamine contamination, FDA has also "asked the Centers for Disease Control and Prevention (CDC) to use its surveillance network to monitor for signs of human illness, such as increased renal failure, that could indicate contamination of the human food supply."

Brief description and background

In 2007 a pet food recall was initiated by Menu Foods and other pet food manufacturers who had found their products had been contaminated and caused serious illnesses or deaths in some of the animals that had eaten them.

On 30 March 2007, the US Food and Drug Administration reported finding white granular melamine in the pet food, in samples of white granular wheat gluten imported from a single source in China, Xuzhou Anying Biologic Technology as well as in crystalline form in the kidneys and in urine of affected animals. Further vegetable protein imported from China was later implicated. See 2007 pet food crisis.

The practice of adding "melamine scrap" to animal feed is reported to be widespread in China in order to give the appearance of increased protein content in animal feed.[37] The presence of melamine has not been conclusively linked to the deaths of animals, as this chemical was previously thought to be relatively non-toxic at low doses; however, now that it is added to the human food chain, taken over time, new sicknesses and even death is not far behind.

CHEMICALS IN FOOD PACKAGING

Dangers of packaging chemicals getting into food

Brief Summary:

Harmful chemicals from plastic or Styrofoam packaging can penetrate the foods, and may cause health problems such as cancer. Plastic wrapping on microwavable foods can transmit the chemicals during heating. Other products packaged with safe materials are discussed.
More than a decade ago, it was discovered that an ordinary Styrofoam cup could disintegrate when it held hot tea and lemon. Discoveries of such unanticipated interactions still occur from time to time.

For many years, polystyrene egg containers have largely replaced papier-mâché. However, their safety has only recently been investigated, in 1991. The Louisiana Agricultural Experiment Station reported that volatile styrene monomers were detected in shell eggs stored in polystyrene containers for two weeks in supermarkets. Egg dishes cooked with these contaminated eggs contained seven times more ethylbenzene and styrene than those prepared from fresh farm eggs that had not been packaged in polystyrene. It is suspected that the volatile compounds can migrate through the porous shells into the edible portions of eggs.

Benzene from multilayer, oxygen-barrier, laminated bags has been found to migrate into meat, poultry, cheeses, and other packaged foods. This problem surfaced in September 1990 when an off-odor was noted in a roast beef shipment. Investigation showed that the meat contained benzene from the packaging, ranging from less than 5 parts per billion (ppb) to 17.8 ppb in raw meat. The benzene volatilized when the meat was heated.

Increasingly, plastic food wraps and containers have gained in popularity for microwaving foods. This practice can release components from the plastics, including base monomers, plasticizers, colorants, and stabilizers, especially when high heat is used. Many plastics contain plasticizers, used to increase the wrap's flexibility. Some plasticizers have been found to migrate from the plastic into food. One is DEHA [di(ethylhexyl)adepate], commonly used as a plasticizer in polyvinyl chloride (PVC) film wrap, which is popular for covering stored and micro-waved food. DEHA is a suspected carcinogen.

In a 1987 study of home use of PVC film wrap, the DEHA migration level was found to increase in proportion to the time that the food was in contact with the PVC wrap and with the rise in cooking temperature. The highest migration levels were found when the plastic film was in direct contact with food with a high fat content on its surface. The highest migration levels were found with micro-waved meats (such as pork, spareribs, and roast chicken), and bakery products (such as cakes, scones, and biscuits made with peanuts). Somewhat lower levels were found in fruits and vegetables, except avocado with its high fat content. Migration levels were low when there was little or no direct contact between the food and the wrap.

In the same study, use of PVC film with foods in retail stores was examined. Results were similar. The amount of DEHA migration into foods depended on how long the film was in contact with fatty surfaces of food. The highest amounts were found in cheeses, baked goods, and sandwiches; lower amounts in cooked meat and poultry; and the lowest, in fruits and vegetables.

Polyethylene, a popular plastic film commonly used for food freezer bags and wraps, does not contain plasticizers, and is considered to be generally safe for microwaving foods. However, if printing has been applied to the surface, the primer applied to the plastic prior to printing, as well as the applied inks, may subject the heated plastic to conditions distinctly different from those for which they had been tested and approved. Only clear polyethylene is suitable for microwaving food.

Formed plastic containers, used for carry-out foods, should not be re-used for microwaving. Such containers, if heated, may be subjected to conditions other than those for which they had been safety tested.

Some plastic packaging materials now in use for microwaving have not been approved for use at high heat. The most severe conditions for such packaging recognized by protocols of the Food and Drug Administration (FDA) were under conditions that previously had prevailed: from 212[degrees]F to 275[degrees]F. Recognizing the changes that have occurred, FDA scientists are working with members of the packaging industry to study new testing procedures, and to learn whether packaging materials can be modified to assure food safety when used for cooking at high heat.

Of concern, too, is "active packaging." Thin layers or strips of metallic heat susceptors are placed in plastic food packaging intended for microwaving. The susceptors focus microwave radiation to produce extremely hot surfaces (400[degrees]F to 500[degrees]F) within the package. This high heat permits food to be browned, crisped, or popped--features usually lacking in microwave cooking. At such high heat, substances such as polymers and their breakdown products, as well as adhesives and their components and other substances present in the plastic, can migrate into the food. Originally, susceptor strips were approved by the FDA for a different purpose, and were tested at far lower temperatures.

Polyethylene terephthalate (PET) is a popular plastic film wrap. It had long been assumed that PET film provides a functional barrier to adhesive components. It was demonstrated recently that the film allowed the migration of adhesive components into foods when oils or foods were cooked in contact with it. A study by the FDA's Division of Food Chemistry and Technology showed that the susceptor board components that migrated in the largest quantities were the plasticizers rather than the polymer components, even though the polymer components were in direct contact with the oil or food, whereas the plasticizers were in the adhesive layer of the susceptor boards. Approximately 50% more plasticizers migrated than did polymer components.

For many years, a purple dye (FD&C Violet No. 1) had been used to stamp inspected meat. The dye was suspected as a carcinogen. There was no assurance that the portion of the meat with the dye would be cut away before being consumed. In 1973, the FDA banned the dye as a meat marker.

Nitrosamines (carcinogenic compounds) were discovered in rubber nipples used to cap baby bottles. The rubber was reformulated to eliminate nitrosame formation. More recently, nitrosamines were discovered in hams that had rubber netting to encase them after boning and curing. The rubber was reformulated to eliminate this problem.

With rapidly changing packaging practices and many innovative techniques, manufacturers and regulators need to be vigilant in order to prevent unanticipated and undesirable interactions with foods.

In 2006, Americans bought more than 4 billion gallons of water in individual-portion bottles. Most of the containers end up in the trash. But now, in the global market for the bottles, once they're recycled, the commercialization train has just left again.
Many water companies choose pristine spots in areas saturated with springs, especially about a decade ago, when the bottled water market was taking off. These companies go to great lengths to protect the watershed. But in order to sell spring water competitively, it bottles the water using a non-renewable resource: **polyethylene terephthalate**, or PET, made from natural gas and petroleum.

Billions of Bottles Born

At times, the plant produces more than 30,000 bottles a minute. They march through the plant single file, knocking into each other like bumper cars before getting filled. This plant produced 1.8 billion bottles of water in 2006. They're made from what is called a "preform," composed of PET resin that is melted and molded. Next, it's heated, stretched and blown out, like a balloon, into a bottle.

Kim Jeffrey, the president and CEO of Nestlé Waters North America, says it was the PET bottle that jump-started the bottled water industry. Poland Spring, one of Nestlé's brands, first bottled water in PET in 1990.

"It revolutionized our industry," Jeffrey says, "because now people could get bottled water in the same format they were getting soft drinks in ... and that changed everything."

Today, consumers can take water on the go. But the bottles don't always get tossed into recycling bins. Only about 23 percent of bottles, including soda, are recycled.

Demand for Recycled Bottles

In Hartford, Conn., trucks transport recycled plastic, glass and aluminum from residents' homes to the Connecticut Resources Recovery Authority, one of hundreds of recycling facilities in the U.S. Sean Duffy is president of Fairfield County Recycling, which operates the plant. He says water bottles collected from the curbside recycling program yield valuable material. Duffy's company makes a profit on each bottle made from PET. "We have the capacity to process it, and it is in high demand," Duffy says. "So we want every pound we can get."

Paul Zordan also wants every pound he can get. Zordan is constantly looking for bottles. He's vice president of UltrePET, a PET "reclaimer" in Albany, N.Y. Reclaiming PET is grimey, grungy work. It begins by sorting through dirty bottles, by machine and by hand. It looks like garbage, but, Zordan says, "It's gonna be money to us if we can do our job right. It's garbage now, but it's going to turn into a usable resin to make something out of."

Hot Market in China

UltrePET cleans the bottles and then chops them into chips, each smaller than a cornflake. Zordan describes his work as mining. Indeed, the white flakes mined from the would-be trash sparkle like diamonds. Then, they're heated and turned into tiny white pellets of recycled PET, which competes on the marketplace with virgin PET. It's a hot market — so hot that the Chinese are coming to the U.S. to buy nearly 40 percent of the bottles Americans recycle.

"China is the No. 1 consumer of the material collected in this country," Zordan says. "So if they're taking the lion's share, then there's only so much available for people like us." While used bottles from the U.S. are going to China, reclaimers like Zordan are criss-crossing the U.S. and even going to Canada, Mexico and Latin America to find PET. In all, they imported nearly 300 million pounds of flakes and bottles in 2005.

Bottle's Afterlife: Your Carpet?

Recycled PET can be made into fiber, and then purchased by companies such as Interface Fabrics in Guilford, Maine.

The company's industrial loom weaves a heathered grey-blue cloth, with a silky finish, that will eventually become the wall covering for office cubicles. Ben King oversees operations for Interface Fabrics.

"We got colors — all different kinds — all on recycled polyester, almost exclusively," he says. "We run a little bit of wool, but almost everything in here is recycled polyester."

Recycled PET is turning up in a lot of items: carpets, clothing, automotive parts and even new bottles. With so much demand for the empties — and so many bottles in the marketplace — the question pressing on recyclers and beverage companies alike is how to get more of them recycled.

Styrofoam Uses: Food and Beverage Containers

Styrofoam, the Dow Chemical brand name for Polystyrene, is perhaps most widely known for its use as coffee cups, disposable plates and take-out containers.

The reasons for its popularity is that it has excellent insulating properties that keep hot products hot and cold products cold much longer than disposable paper cups and boxes.

Styrofoam Uses: Food and Beverage Containers

Here is a list of the different uses for polystyrene products related to our food.

- Cups.

- Plates.
- Utensils (un-blown polystyrene).
- Take-out boxes.
- Egg cartons.
- Clear plastic cups and boxes (un-blown polystyrene).

Styrofoam Uses: Packaging Products

Using pre-molded Styrofoam or "peanuts" for packing delicate objects is probably the other most commonly known of use for this material.

For a long time, Styrofoam was the best packing material being light-weight and protective at the same time. However, in the past decade large, inflated air sacs have gained popularity as an even cheaper and effective packing material because it uses air and very few resources to create.

Styrofoam Uses: Packaging Products

Most Styrofoam packaging is either the little popcorn-like pieces referred to as "peanuts" or the large molded piece to fit a specific product.

If you ever come across packaging that looks like cut-up odd pieces of Styrofoam, it is re-used molded pieces that have been shredded down.

In the same way that the FDA monitors additives in foods, it also monitors packaging that comes in contact with food for transporting, storing or cooking. Manufacturers are required by law to obtain approval from the FDA for all materials used in food packages before they can be marketed.

Sometimes people use food packages for purposes other than FDA-regulated uses — for example, some people will turn bread bags inside out and reuse them to store food or pack lunches. The FDA strongly advises against such use because of the possible risk of lead contamination from the ink on the outside of the bread bag, or contamination from dirty hands, insects or bacteria from other contacts.

Microwave-safe Containers:

Consumers are advised not to use plastic containers, which were not intended for microwave use, in the microwave. This would include margarine tubs, whipped topping bowls and cheese containers that can warp or melt from hot food, possibly causing chemical migration. Remove food from store wrap prior to microwave defrosting. Foam trays and plastic wraps are not heat stable at high temperatures. Melting or warping from hot food may cause chemicals to migrate into food. Avoid letting any plastic wraps or thin plastic storage bags touch foods during microwaving. Never use brown grocery bags or newspapers in the microwave.

Aluminum

Even though aluminum is not considered to be a heavy metal like lead, it can be toxic in excessive amounts and even in small amounts if it is deposited in the brain. Many of the symptoms of aluminum toxicity mimic those of Alzheimer's disease and osteoporosis. Colic, rickets, gastrointestinal problems, interference with the metabolism of calcium, extreme nervousness, anemia, headaches, decreased liver and kidney function, memory loss, speech problems, softening of the bones, and aching muscles can all be caused by aluminum toxicity.

Aluminum is excreted by the kidneys, therefore toxic amounts can impair kidney function. Aluminum can also accumulate in the brain causing seizures and reduced mental alertness. The brain is normally protected by a blood-brain barrier, which filters the blood before it reaches it. Elemental aluminum does not pass easily through this barrier, but certain compounds contained within aluminum, such as aluminum fluoride do. Interestingly, many municipal water supplies are treated with both aluminum sulfate and aluminum fluoride. These two chemicals can also combine easily in the blood. Aluminum fluoride is also poorly excreted in the urine.

When there is a high level of absorption of aluminum and silicon, the combination can result in an accumulation of certain compounds in the cerebral cortex and can prevent nerve impulses being carried to and from the brain properly. Long term calcium deficiency can further aggravate the condition. Workers in aluminum smelting plants on a long term basis, have been know to experience dizziness, poor coordination, balance problems and tiredness. It has been claimed that the accumulation of aluminum in the brain could be a possible cause for these issues.

It is estimated that the normal person takes in between 3 and 10 milligrams of aluminum per day. Aluminum is the most abundant metallic element produced by the earth. It can be absorbed into the body through the digestive tract, the lungs and the skin, and is also absorbed by and accumulates in the bodies tissues. Aluminum is found naturally in our air, water and soil. It is also used in the process of making cooking pots and pans, utensils and foil. Other items such as over the counter pain killers, anti-inflammatory products, and douche preparations can also contain aluminum. Aluminum is also an additive in most baking powders, is used in food processing, and is present in antiperspirants, toothpaste, dental amalgams, bleached flour, grated cheese, table salt, and beer, (especially when the beer is in aluminum cans). The biggest source of aluminum, however, comes from our municipal water supplies.

Excessive use of antacids is also a common cause of aluminum toxicity in this country, especially for those who have kidney problems. Many over the counter type antacids contain amounts of aluminum hydroxide that may be too much for the kidneys to handle properly.

So, what can we do to prevent aluminum toxicity from happening to ourselves and our families?

1. Eat a diet that is high in fiber and includes apple pectin.

2. Use stainless steel, glass, or iron cookware. Stainless steel is a good choic.

3. Beware of any productcontaining aluminum or dihydroxyaluminum.

4. A hair analysis can be used to determine levels of aluminum in the body.

5. Research has shown that the longer you cook food in aluminum pots, the more they corrode, and the more aluminum is absorbed into the food and hence into the body. Aluminum is more readily dissolved by acid forming foods, such as coffee, cheese, meat, black and green tea, cabbage, cucumbers, tomatoes, turnips, spinach and radishes.

6. Acid rain leeches aluminum out of the soil and into drinking water.

Dangers of Aluminum Toxicity

Autopsies on a large amount of people who have died of Alzheimer's disease showed accumulations of up to four times the normal amount of aluminum in the nerve cells in the brain, especially in the hippocampus which plays a central role in memory.

Products To Avoid

Aluminum Cookware

A study done by the University of Cincinnati Medical Center showed that using aluminum pots and pans to cook tomatoes doubled the aluminum content of the tomatoes, from 2 to 4 milligrams per serving.

Antacids

Many name brand antacids contain aluminum hydroxide.

Aluminum free antacids are also available such as Alka-Seltzer, Alka Mints, Di-Gel tablets, Maalox caplets, Mylanta gel caps, Rolaids tablets, Titralac, and Tums E-X.

Antidiarrheal Products

Watch labels carefully for any mention of aluminum salts.

Products containing loperamide such as Imodium AD usually do not contain aluminum salts.

Buffered Aspirin

Buffered aspirin can contain up to 14.4 to 88 milligrams of aluminum hydroxide or aluminum glycinate. Ordinary aspirin is aluminum free as are many other pain killers.

Containers

Aluminum coated waxed containers, used especially for orange and pineapple juices, cause juices inside to absorb aluminum. Beer and soft drinks that are stored in aluminum cans also absorb small quantities of aluminum. Bottled beverages are better.

Deodorants

Many deodorants and antiperspirants and even some skin powders contain aluminum chlorhydrate. Aluminum in this form is more readily absorbed into the brain via the nasal passages.

Douches

Many popular douche products contain aluminum salts. A homemade version of vinegar and water can be substituted.

Food Additives

Cake mixes, frozen doughs, self-rising flour, and sliced process cheese food all contain from 5 to 50 milligrams of sodium aluminum phosphate per average serving. Baking powder has 5 to 70 milligrams of sodium aluminum sulfate per teaspoon. Starch modifiers and anti caking agents also contain varying levels of aluminum compounds. The processed cheeses used on cheese burgers at fast food restaurants also contain aluminum, which is added to make the cheese melt better.

Shampoos

A number of anti-dandruff preparations contain magnesium aluminum silicate. Watch labels carefully for aluminum lauryl sulfate, which is a common ingredient in many popular shampoo products.

This information is for informational purpose only and is not intended to replace the care or advice of a physician.

PESTICIDES

If you have a garden, you know the serious toll that pests, diseases and weeds can take on your backyard harvest. Each year, as much as 45 percent of the world's crops are lost to damage or spoilage. Careful and judicious use of pesticides can minimize these losses, help produce a safe and abundant food supply, and keep a variety of fruits, vegetables, breads and other foods on your table year-round at affordable prices.

What Are Pesticides?

Pesticides are a group of chemicals designed to control weeds, diseases, insects or other pests on crops, landscape plants or animals. The most commonly used pesticides are insecticides (to control insects), fungicides (to control fungi) and herbicides (to control weeds). Prudent use of pesticides has played a vital role in feeding the world's growing population by dramatically increasing crop yields.

Who Approves the Use of Pesticides?

The U.S. Environmental Protection Agency (EPA) is charged by law with regulating the development, distribution, use and disposal of pesticides. Before approving or registering a pesticide for use in growing food, the EPA can require more than 120 different tests — depending on the uses of the pesticide — to determine its safety. The agency registers only those pesticides that meet their standards for human health, the environment and wildlife. If new research shows that any registered pesticide does not meet their standards, the EPA will cancel or modify its use.

How Does the EPA Regulate Pesticide Use?

When approving a pesticide, the EPA specifies instructions for its use on the label, which must be followed by law. The agency also establishes a tolerance for each pesticide it approves. A tolerance is the maximum residue level of a pesticide legally permitted in or on a food. A tolerance ensures that, when pesticides are used according to label directions, the remaining pesticide residues will not pose an unacceptable health risk to anyone — from infants to adults — who consumes the food.

Tolerances are considered an enforcement tool and are used by the FDA in its monitoring program to ensure a safe food supply. If any pesticide residue is found to exceed its tolerance on a food, then the food is not permitted to be sold.

The Food Quality Protection Act, signed into law in 1996, now sets an even tougher standard for pesticide use on food. The EPA will consider the public's overall exposure to pesticides (through food, water and in home environments) when making decisions to set standards for pesticide use on food. These new standards are especially intended to protect infants and children who may be more vulnerable to pesticide exposure.

SOLVENTS

Petroleum/Petrolatum

What is petroleum?

Crude oil, sometimes called petroleum, is a fossil fuel that was produced deep in the earth through a process that took millions of years to complete.

Millions of years later, almost all of us come into contact with a derivative of petroleum every day. Through a process called fractional distillation, petroleum refineries break petroleum into many of its smaller components. Each of these smaller components is made up of molecules called hydrocarbons.

The world is full of products that come from petroleum. For example, gasoline, styrofoam, lubricating oils, and many other items are all derivatives of this raw material. How are petroleum and cosmetics related? The two seemingly unrelated items, petroleum and cosmetics, are indeed closely related in our modern world.

Mineral oil and petroleum are the basic ingredients in many cosmetic products today. Both mineral oil and petroleum have the same origins in fossils fuels. Cosmetics such as foundations, cleansers, and moisturizers often contain mineral oil. By locking moisture against the skin, mineral oil sits on the skin's surface and can potentially block pores. This may cause the appearance of pimples because the skin cannot properly 'breathe'.

Fragrances in lotions, shampoos, and many other cosmetic products are composed of aromatic hydrocarbons. Perfumes and products containing fragrance can contain many hundreds of chemicals to produce a distinct scent. A significant number of these aromas are derived from petroleum.

One popular chemical additive that carries moisture in cosmetics is propylene glycol. It is also a derivative of petroleum. Some products that list propylene glycol as an ingredient include:

anti-freeze
laundry detergent
paint
shampoo
conditioner

Past research links propylene glycol to serious health problems as liver and kidney damage as well as respiratory irritation or nausea if swallowed.

An antiseptic, isopropyl alcohol, kills bacteria on the skin. You can find it on the ingredient list of cleansers, toners and other cosmetic products. Unfortunately, this derivative of petroleum dries the skin and may cause miniature cracks in the skin that allow bacteria to enter, potentially causing irritations or pimples.

Do these petroleum-derived products affect your health?

Your skin covers your body and acts as a physical barrier to many of the pollutants in the atmosphere. When you use products on your skin such as cosmetics, lotions, and shampoos, the ingredients in these products come into direct contact with your body's largest organ; your skin. You may ask yourself, where do the ingredients in the products go? Modern research at the Herb Research Foundation found that the skin absorbs up to 60% of the chemicals in products that it comes into contact with directly into the bloodstream. Today, hormone therapy treatments and smoking cessation medications are often prescribed as patches that you apply directly to the skin. The medication passes through the skin and directly enters the bloodstream.

Cosmetics

For pregnant women, the risk is not only for her body but also for the developing fetus. If the chemicals found in cosmetics readily enter the bloodstream when applied to the skin, then they will also reach the developing baby. Researchers at the Brunel University in England are looking closely at a family of preservatives called parabens. Their research has recently linked parabens to the possibility that male babies will have lower sperm counts. These preservatives are derived from petroleum and help to maintain the freshness and integrity of the product. Currently, many manufacturers add parabens to cosmetics to allow a minimum of 3 years shelf life. Therefore, the parabens kill any bacteria that could potentially enter the product. If these chemical ingredients can kill the bacterial cells, what are they doing to your skin cells? In most cases, there is no conclusive answer to this question. However, the research mentioned strongly suggests that the synthetic ingredients may have a significant impact on our bodies.

In many cases, the long-term effects of many of the chemical additives in our cosmetics are not known. However, other chemical additives are known carcinogens. These types of chemicals can cause cancer in humans. Such chemicals include some artificial colors in cosmetics. The effects of chemicals and other synthetic ingredients in cosmetics may lead to mild allergic reactions causing rashes and minor skin irritation to more significant problems such as lesions on the skin.

Cologne, Perfumes, & Oil Fragrances

You spray your favorite perfume as you get ready for the new day. You want to start off smelling great but you might not know that you could actually be harming yourself or others in your household with each spritz. Are you wondering how something that smells as wonderful as your perfume could be harmful? The answer to this question may be surprising.

Chemicals can cause several different types of health problems; most everyone knows this and we limit our exposure to chemicals as much as possible. What people don't seem to realize is that each time you spray yourself with a squirt of perfume, you are spraying chemicals directly on your body and into the air around you. After all, it takes chemicals to make perfumes.

These compounds are called fragrance chemicals and they vaporize when sprayed into the air or on your skin. As you and others around you breathe in these scents you are being exposed to chemicals that may be harmful.

Anywhere that perfumes are used the quality of the air is affected. These fragrance chemicals are not only found in perfumes and colognes, but also in scented candles, incense sticks, vaporizers and fragrance oils. When you use these fragrances inside your home the indoor air quality is greatly reduced.

Problems Caused by Perfumes

Do you have a lot of problems with allergies? Does your nose feel so stopped up all the time that taking sinus medication has became a regular routine? If your answer is yes, do you or someone in your home use perfume on a regular basis? If so, it is possible that this could be your main problem. An estimated 2% of the population in developed countries suffers with some form of fragrance allergy.

Being exposed to fragrances can cause many problems, including but not limited to the ones listed below.

- Sinusitis
- Headaches
- Nose and throat irritation
- Eye irritation
- Loss of coordination
- Defects of the central nervous system
- Birth defects
- Forgetfulness
- Cancer

Of course, not everyone has these problems when exposed to perfumes. Neither does one person have all of these symptoms listed above, but you could be suffering with some of these problems and not know that it is being caused from a fragrance. Just as some people experience an allergic reaction to some foods, others are allergic to fragrances. Some ingredients that are found in these alluring aromas can even cause someone with asthma to suffer from an increased amount of asthma attacks. If you find that you are suffering with a lot of sinus problems see how many different scents you are exposed to each day.

If you are like most people you probably never thought that something as simple as a bottle of perfume or scented candle could cause so many serious problems. Your first thought would most likely be how could something that smells so nice cause you to be forgetful or even cause cancer.

Unfortunately, there is a danger and the more fragrant chemicals you are exposed to each day increase this danger. Just think about how many different perfumes the average person is exposed to on a daily basis. At work, restaurants, stores, school. Everywhere you go someone has on his or her favorite perfume and you are constantly breathing in all these different chemicals each day.

Information about Perfume Ingredients

All kinds of fragrances can be created with modern technology. If you can name it, you can smell it. Perfumed oils to extravagant designer perfumes are being developed on a regular basis.

Everything from cheap perfumes to expensive name brands can be purchased easily and most people never think twice about what they are made from.

Currently there are upwards of 800 different fragrance chemicals and oils used in perfumes and scented candles.

Unfortunately, manufacturers in many countries are not required to state exactly what ingredients make up a certain fragrance; they are considered a trade secret.

Added to this, over half of the ingredients used in perfumes have never been tested to see how toxic they are to humans. Therefore, few studies have been done to see how they affect the average person's health, especially when exposed to the chemicals for a long period of time. However, when we consider how some scented candles contain carbon monoxide, acetone, lead or benzene it's not difficult to imagine how mixing a bunch of different chemicals together could affect our health.

Perfumes can have as little as one ingredient to hundreds of fragrant ingredients in any one brand.

However, out of the ingredients that have been tested at least a fourth of the fragrance chemicals have been found to contain toxic substances. It is not just man made fragrances that have adverse side effects on people but natural ingredients have also been found to be harmful.

Below is a list of natural fragrances that research has proven to be harmful. Please be aware if these are in your perfume or cologne.

- Orris root
- Patchouli oil
- Galbanum
- Civet
- Bergamot
- Asafetida

If you already have sensitive skin, asthma, or any other respiratory problem perfumes will affect you even more than the average healthy person. However, a healthy person can begin to experience hypersensitivity to perfumes over a period of time. One of the most obvious signs of having a reaction to a particular fragrance is developing a rash. If you do notice a rash after using a product discontinue immediately, no matter how slight it may be.

Sometimes a chemical used to create a specific scent may have a very unpleasant smell to it. In these cases another fragrance is normally used to cover that smell up, but covering the smell does not eliminate it. These odors can still be harmful to people who breathe them, even though you can not smell the harmful odor.

Chemicals enter your body through breathing or through your skin. Each time you breathe in the scent of perfume you run the risk of exposing yourself to harmful fragrances. Each time you apply perfume to your skin it penetrates the skin and soaks into the body's tissues. Over time this can even begin to affect internal organs.

Women's perfumes are not the only ones that contain harmful chemicals; men's cologne also poses the same problem.

In the case of scented candles, fragrance oils and incense sticks, these pose a particular danger when lit. The perfume fragrance is then released by a chemical reaction with the burning wick to release these chemicals into the air, which we then take into our lungs.

This can produce headaches, sickness, cause breathing difficulties and irritate the ear, nose and throat.

Now, here is the good news. Ever since research began showing that fragrances can be harmful, changes have been made to make perfumes safer to use. In some countries manufacturers are obliged to detail the fragrance ingredients so the end user can make informed choices.

What are your alternatives for cosmetics?

Luckily, there are alternatives to cosmetics filled with synthetically produced ingredients. Increasingly, cosmetic manufacturers are answering the public's demand for alternatives to the chemically loaded beauty and grooming supplies. The Organic Make-up Company is one such company that is leading the way in producing high-quality, organically manufactured cosmetics! As a consumer, you have the ability to decrease the number of preservatives and chemical additives your skin comes into contact with and therefore, that may enter your body. To avoid using the synthetically derived fragrances, look for products containing essential oils. These are pure oils derived from flowers and other plants in nature.

All you have to do is make the simple choice of purchasing cosmetic products with all-natural, organic ingredients. Whether you continue using cosmetics that contain petroleum-based ingredients or not is a personal choice. What is most important is to get the facts and to know that you have a choice when it comes to buying organic or synthetic cosmetic products. See our site links in the rear of this book.

BENZENE

What is benzene?

Benzene, also known as benzol, is a colorless liquid with a sweet odor, and can be described as a volatile organic compound. The chemical symbol for benzene is C6H6.

Benzene is formed from both natural processes and human activities. It is produced from volcanoes and forest fires, and is a natural part of crude oil, gasoline, and cigarette smoke.

Benzene is one of the 20 most widely used chemicals in the United States. It is used to make other chemicals that are then used to make plastics, resins, nylon, and other synthetic fibers. It is used to make explosives, photographic chemicals, rubber, lubricants, dyes, adhesives, coatings, paint, detergents, drugs, and pesticides. It is used in printing, lithography, and food processing. It has been used as a gasoline additive in the past, but that use has been greatly reduced in the United States since the 1990s.

How might I be exposed to benzene?

Benzene is found in the air, water, and soil. You can be exposed to small amounts of benzene outdoors, where the air can contain low levels from tobacco smoke, automotive service stations, vehicle exhaust, and industrial emissions. You can be exposed to higher levels of benzene near gas stations, hazardous waste sites, or industrial facilities.

You can be exposed to benzene indoors at home, where the air can contain higher levels of benzene than outdoor air, from products such as glue, paint, furniture wax, and detergent.

Approximately half the national exposure to benzene comes from smoking cigarettes or being exposed to cigarette smoke, indoors or outdoors. You can be exposed to benzene by drinking or using well water that has been contaminated by leaking underground gasoline storage tanks or hazardous waste sites, though those levels are usually less than those from industrial facilities and smoking cigarettes.

You can be exposed to higher than normal levels of benzene at work if you work at a facility that makes or uses benzene, including petroleum refining sites, pharmaceutical plants, petrochemical manufacturing facilities, rubber tire manufacturing facilities, or gas stations. You may be exposed if you are a steel worker, printer, shoemaker, laboratory technician, or firefighter.

How can benzene affect my health?

Benzene is classified as a carcinogen by the National Toxicology Program because it has been known to cause cancer. Long-term exposure to high levels of benzene can cause leukemia.

Breathing very high levels of benzene, or eating or drinking foods contaminated with high levels of benzene, can cause death. Eating or drinking foods contaminated with high levels of benzene can also cause vomiting and stomach irritation. Small amounts of benzene, which are not harmful, can be found in fruit, fish, vegetables, nuts, dairy products, beverages, and eggs.

Short-term exposure to high levels of benzene by breathing or eating affects the central nervous system, and can cause paralysis, coma, convulsions, dizziness, sleepiness, rapid heart rate, tightness of the chest, tremors, and rapid breathing.

If you work at a facility that uses benzene, breathing high levels of benzene can cause irreversible brain damage, unconsciousness, cardiac arrest, blurred vision, headaches, tremors, confusion, and fatigue. In women, it can shrink ovaries and cause menstrual irregularity. Spilling benzene on your skin can cause redness, sores, scaling, and drying of the skin. If benzene contacts the eyes, it can cause irritation and damage to the cornea.

Long-term exposure to benzene can decrease red blood cells, leading to anemia. It can also cause excessive bleeding and affect the immune system, increasing the chance of infection.

BENZENE POLLUTED PRODUCTS (Throw These Out)

(Your health is worth more than the fortune you spent on them!)

- Flavored food, yogurt, candies, throat lozenges, store-bought cookies, cakes
- Cooking oil and shortening (use only olive oil, and butter
- Beverages including bottled water, and store bought fruit juice
- Toothpaste, including health brands
- Cold cereal, including health brands
- Ice cream and frozen yogurt
- Hand cream, skin cream, moisturizers
- Chewing gum
- Petroleum Jelly products (skin cream TM, Lip Therapy TM), chap stick, hand cleaners
- Vitamins and other health supplements, unless tested
- Personal lubricant, including lubricated condoms
- Tea Tree oil products (except the one shown)
- Cattle and poultry feeds, except simple grains
- Flavored pet food, both for cats and dogs
- Bird food made into cake

Propylene Alcohol

- Isopropyl Alcohol can affect you when breathed in and by passing through your skin.
- Contact can irritate and burn the skin and eyes. Repeated skin exposure can cause itching, redness, rash, drying and cracking.
- Breathing Isopropyl Alcohol can irritate the nose and throat.
- Overexposure can cause headache, drowsiness, confusion, loss of coordination, unconsciousness and death.
- Isopropyl Alcohol may affect the liver and kidneys.
- Isopropyl Alcohol is a FLAMMABLE LIQUID and a FIRE HAZARD.

IDENTIFICATION

Isopropyl Alcohol is a colorless liquid. It is used as a solvent and in making many commercial products. Rubbing Alcohol is a solution containing Isopropyl Alcohol.

REASON FOR CITATION

Isopropyl Alcohol is on the Hazardous Substance List because it is regulated by OSHA and cited by ACGIH, DOT, NIOSH, DEP, NFPA and EPA.\

PROPYLENE ALCOHOL POLLUTED PRODUCTS

THROW THESE OUT!
(even if it is not listed on the label!)

- shampoo
- hair spray and mousse
- cold cereals, even natural granolas
- cosmetics, addressed below
- mouthwash
- decaffenianted coffee, PostumTM, herb tea blends (single herb teas ok)
- Vitamins, minerals and supplements
- Bottled water, distilled water or spring
- Rubbing alcohol
- White sugar
- All shaving supplies including aftershave
- Carbonated beverages
- Store-bought fruit juices, including health food bran

PARASITES & POLLUTION

Everything living on you or in you, not just setting on you, but takes its food from you, regardless of its size, is a parasite.

Big worms need to be distinguished from the medium - sized amoebae, the even smaller bacteria and the smallest of all viruses. Although the term parasite is usually reserved for bigger worms, we will use the word parasite for all sizes. No matter what its size, it can be called a parasite.

Parasitic worms come in different shapes and go through stages of development that can look very, very different from the adult: roundworms and flatworms. Roundworms are round similar to earthworms even though they may be as thin as paper like Trichinella, which is found in pork especially. There are other thin worms as well such as threadworms, filarial or microscopically. Flatworms are more like leeches. They generally attach themselves with the head (scolex) like tapeworms, commonly with a special sucker like flukes.

Roundworms like common cat and dog roundworm, are simplest. The eggs are swallowed by licking or eating a bit of filth. They hatch into a tiny larva. The larva treks to the

lungs. You cough it up and swallow it. Meanwhile it has shedded periodically part or all of a coat or an outer covering a few times. It then crawls to the intestine where it becomes an adult, shedding eggs in your stool.
Worms usually have preferred locations. The favorite organ for Dirofilaria, A genus of filarial worms including the heartworm and other species or a dog heartworm, is the heart usually found in mammals other than humans. Sometimes the rules can be broken. Tests have shown that Dirofilaria can live in other organs, too, if there are sufficiently polluted solvents, metals and toxins.

Flatworms like tapeworms are much more complicated in their life history. You could eat the eggs accidentally with dirt, or ingesting anything with these microscopic eggs on it. After hatching, the tiny larva burrows into its favorite organ. Your body encases it with a cyst. The white blood cells have been taught never to attack your body...and the cyst case is your body! So the tapeworm stage has safe residence for some time. If you are a meat eater, you could eat such a cyst if it happens to be lodged in the meat you are eating! Your teeth break it apart as you crunch. The little larva is swallowed and tries to attach itself to your intestine with its head. Then it grows longer by making segment after segment. The segments with their eggs leave with the bowel contents. Often dog tapeworm of the small variety are found on the animal's human owner.

Flatworms like flukes are also very complicated. The eggs, passed out with bowel contents are not meant to be eaten as such. They are meant to hatch in ponds where snails and minnows eat them. The larva grows up in these new "secondary" hosts. Later, the snail sheds them and they attach themselves to foliage near the pond. Over the course of winter, they are incased in a tough metacercarial cyst. An unsuspecting browsing animal now eats them. They come out of their metacercarial cyst as a small adult and quickly attach themselves to the intestine with a sucker. They now have "safe haven" and can go about maturing and laying eggs.

There are four common flukes that are found in humans: human intestinal fluke, human liver fluke, sheep liver fluke, pancreatic fluke of cattle.

The Worst Parasite

The **Fasciolopsis buskii fluke or flatworm** is found in every case of cancer, HIV infection, Alzheimer's, Crohn's disease, Kaposi's, endometriosis, and in many people without these diseases. There are six different stages in its life cycle:

The adult is the only stage that "normally" lives in the human and then only in the intestine. Fasciolopsis depends on a snail, called a secondary host, for part of its life cycle. But when your body has solvents, such as regular house alcohol, cologne, perfume, after shave, for example, the other five stages can develop in you as well!

If proply alcohol is the solvent, which is in thousands of household products from body lotion to shampoo, the intestinal fluke is invited to use another organ as a secondary host - this organ will become cancerous. If benzene is the solvent, which comes in the form of soft drinks, bottled drinking water, and store-bought fruit juices, to name a few, the intestinal fluke uses the thymus for its secondary host, setting the stage for AIDS. Wood alcohol, which comes in the form of carbonated drinks, diet drinks, herb tea blends, infant formula, invites pancreatic flukes to use the pancreas as a secondary host. This leads to pancreatic dysfunction, which we call diabetes. If xylene, which comes in the form of carbonated drinks (toluene) are the solvents, at least four flukes use the brain as a secondary host. If methyl ethyl ketone (MEK) or methyl butyl ketone (MBK) are the solvents, which comes in the form of flavored foods, the uterus becomes a secondary host and endometriosis is a likely result.

This is a new kind of characteristic behavior or mode of existence of a parasite or parasitic population, based on pollution. In short, modern food and chemical processes have produced solvent residue that gives the stages of fluke worms the ability to attach themselves to different organs as secondary hosts; thus, setting up diseases that are new. This is why there are so many new diseases popping out of the wood work every day. The interesting thing is that the doctors, hospitals and pharmaceutical companies are already set with their knives, rooms and medicine.

Pollution

Pollutants are all the dead things around us that should not get into your body, because they interfere with its work. They can invade your body via the air you breath, the foods and beverages you eat, and the products you put on your skin, but as long as they don't penetrate your tissues, they won't interfere, like plastic eyeglasses and clothing; yet if they do, your body must fight to remove them.

Pollutants

One of the greatest false assumptions to recognizing pollutants is misdiagnosing the harmful affects. Just because it doesn't "hurt" or a reaction is not detected doesn't mean harm hasn't occurred. One may have escaped an allergic reaction (rash for example) only because they had a stronger immune system. The immune system is like money, paid out of the bank vault for every toxic invasion. When the money is gone, the bank, your health, fails.

Solvent Pollution

Solvents are compounds that dissolve things. Water is a useful, life giving solvent. Most other solvents dissolve fats and are life threatening, because fats form the membrane wall around each of our cells, especially our nerve cells.

The solvent that does the most harm is benzene, as pointed out earlier. It goes to the thymus, ruins our immune system, and causes AIDS. The next worst solvent is propyl alcohol. It goes to the liver and causes cancer in some distant organ. Other major culprits of disease are sylene, toluene, wood alcohol, methylene chloride, and trichloroethane (TCE).

Here are a few Benzene polluted products:

Metal Pollution

Copper from natural sources is essential; however, Inorganic copper, like you would get from a copper bottomed kettle, or many of the newer cooking utencils and cookware may cause cancer. Unfortunately, the inorganic form of metals is what pervades our environment. We put metal jewelry on our skin, eat bread baked in metal pans, and drink water from metal plumbing.

But the worst metallic threat is tooth fillings, which is discussed in more detail on pages 168 – 170.

Mercury amalgam fillings, despite the assurances of the American Dental Association, are not safe. And sometimes the mercury is polluted with thallium, even more toxic than mercury! Gold and silver seem to have fewer harmful effects, but no one should have any pure metal in or on their body.

Other prevalent toxic metals include lead and cadmium from soldered and galvanized plumbing, nickel and chromium from dental ware and cosmetics, and aluminum (see Chemicals in Food Packaging) from the aluminum silicate added to salt to make it run free.

Mycotoxins

Molds produce some of the most toxic substances known called mycotoxins. One small moldy fruit or vegetable can pollute a huge batch of juice, jam or other product. Mycotoxins are not alive, and must be detoxified by your liver.

But because mycotoxins are so extremely poisonous, a tiny amount can incapacitate a part of the liver for days!

Aflatoxin is the most common mycotoxin. It is produced by molds that grow on quite a variety of plants. For that reason eat only perfect citrus fruit, and never drink commercial fruit juice. Of the thousands of oranges that go into the batch of orange juice you drink, one is sure to be moldy, and that is all it takes to give your liver a setback.

A heavy dose of vitamin C helps the liver recover quickly. It also helps get rid of aflatoxin before it is consumed, right in the food container. So keep a plastic shaker of vitamin C powder handy and use it like salt on all your food.

Physical Toxins

Breathing in dust is quite bad for you so your body rejects it by sneezing, coughing, spitting up and out. Imagine breathing in broken glass particles. They cut into the lungs in a thousand places and couldn't be coughed up. They would travel. Imagine swallowing a needle or open pin. If the tip was blunt it could move through the intestine. But because it is sharp it gets caught in your tissue, then works its way deeper and deeper.

If only your body could stop its movement, the harm would be stopped. So your body surrounds it with tough fibrous material so not even a sharp point can get out. Your delicate organs are saved by this protective cyst. But breathing in thousands of microscopic bits of broken glass would require very many cysts. Instead they enlarge to accommodate more and more glass. Now they may be called tumors, although still benign!

Would we ever knowingly breathe in broken glass? We are justifiably afraid of it in our food or under our bare feet. We are unaware that it fills our homes when fiberglass insulation is left imperfectly sealed off. Any hole made through the ceiling or wall, even if covered with cloth, lets swarms of broken glass bits into the house air. Air currents flow inward, into your living space. So all holes leading to insulated spaces must be sealed airtight. Of course, fiberglass should never be used in home construction. The best advice is to have it all removed while you are away and then vacuum and dust.

Occasional exposures by house builders working outdoors does much less harm. Chronic exposure from a single small hole in the ceiling does a lot of harm, leading to cyst formation. And that cyst is a perfect place for parasites and bacteria to settle and multiply. When the intestinal fluke settles there it becomes malignant!

Cancer patients with solid tumors have either fiberglass or asbestos in them.

Asbestos is another tiny bit, sharp as glass, that moves through your body like a swordfish, impaling your cells until it, too, gets routed into a cyst.

We have been led to believe that we no longer have asbestos in our homes because we have outlawed the fireproofing materials it was used in. While that may be true, sources found most often is all too prevalent: the clothes dryer belt. As it gets hot the belt releases a blast of asbestos particles that are forced through the seams of your dryer, and also openings in your exhaust hose, by the high pressure formed inside. It is now in your air.

Chemical Toxins

Chlorofluorocarbons (CFC's) or freon is the refrigerant in your air conditioner and refrigerator coils. CFC's are suspected of causing the ozone hole above the South Pole. All cancer sufferers test positive for CFC's in their cancerous organ! It has been reported that preliminary evidence has shown that it is CFC's that attract other pollutants-fiberglass, metals, PCB's-to form a growing tumor instead of allowing their excretion. This would make it a "super carcinogen.". How could you detect CFC's leaking in your home? By the time your air conditioner or refrigerator needs recharging, you have been exposed for a long time. We desperately need an inexpensive, in home test for this unsuspected killer.

Arsenic is used in pesticide. Why would we poison ourselves along with the cockroaches? Is it because we can't see it happening. It is just as we couldn't see the fiberglass floating in the air? Our diligent scientists have studied the mechanism of arsenic poisoning in great detail. Then why are we allowed to put it on our lawns to be carried into our carpets via shoes?

Polychlorinated biphenyls (PCBs), oily compounds with wonderfully useful electrical properties, were originally used in transformers until their inability to break down into less toxic substances in our environment was spotlighted. Banned from use, they are found in most commercial soap and detergents! Is transformer oil being disposed of by selling it to soap makers?

Formaldehyde is used to cure foam. As a result, foam furniture, pillows and mattresses give off formaldehyde for about two years after manufacturing. If you sleep with your nose buried in a new foam pillow all night, you are risking major lung problems.

Every cleanser in your house probably has a toxic warning on its label. Every fluid your automobile uses is toxic. Every pesticide, herbicide and fertilizer you put on your lawn is probably toxic. Every paint, varnish, wax, lubricant, bleach and detergent will send you to the hospital if even a small amount is ingested. Why do we keep them around?

HOW TO HEAL

"There is no way for us to learn the right way to eat in order to live a long life, except through the guidance and teachings of God.

"The Bible says that He will give us more life abundantly, but He demands strict obedience to His Will. There is no way of prolonging the life of human beings – or any other life – unless it begins with restrictions of the foods which sustain life: the right kinds of food and the proper time when it should be taken into our bodies.

"God has taught His Messengers and prophets how to eat in order to live, but we often become negligent and fall victim to our own negligence. As a result, we call the doctor or go to the hospital, because we did not eat the right foods or in the proper way."

Between negligence and circumstances, we find ours in physically degraded positions needing intensive recuperative care to repair the body's damage and restore it to a level where simple day-to-day eating and maintenance will be sufficient to live healthy.

Your body has been trying to rid itself of its parasites and pollutants all your life! It had its own ways. It made stones; it made mucus secretions; it made itself toxic dumpsites. These were good tactics, but now of course, they are no longer necessary. Can you help your body get rid of these accumulations and sweep itself clean again?

Sweeping your liver clean is the most powerful way of helping your body to heal itself after the parasites are gone. There are thousands of bits of "trash" accumulated in the liver bile ducts. They will turn into stones (gallstones) if left in place.

The kidney, too, has made numerous small stones in its effort to keep your body clear of lead, cadmium, mercury and other impassable pollutants. You can assist the kidney to expel all these.

In days, not weeks or months, you can feel the healing effects of clearing gallstones and kidney stones from your body. But there are miles of bile ducts (50,000 ducts) in the liver, the herbal recipes that do this are used over and over, patiently, until all the "trash" is removed. This can take several years.

So, although you can stop your disease very quickly from progressing, the healing process may not be complete for years.

Nevertheless, you are healthy again. This means your pains are either gone or greatly reduced. Your organs are functioning better. You have a new sense of well-being. Your energy is up. Your desire to live and accomplish something is back.

Killing parasites, removing pollutants and clearing gallstones and kidney stones from your body is a powerful combination of treatments. It is so powerful you can change yourself into a new person in half a year. And then go on improving for years more.

Our objective here is to offer solutions to cleansing yourself of parasites and pollutants for the purpose of eventually coming to a stage of simple day-to-day eating according to the way God prescribes.

THE ROAD TO RECUPERATION

To review our new understanding of health vs. disease:

We have only two problems: parasites and pollutants. Parasites are things that live on us, using up our food and giving us their wastes. Pollutants are toxic things in us making it difficult for our organs to do their work. These two things are responsible for all our other problems. As the Messenger teaches, food could keep us here and food can take us away. We are what we eat.

Our bodies have been trying to rid us of these by making stones, making secretions, giving us swellings, inflammations and benign tumors. We develop deficiencies and disabilities.

Our strategy to undo all this will be a logical one.

- First, we will kill all parasites, bacteria, viruses and fungi.
- Second, we will remove the toxic molds, metals and chemicals in our foods and body products.
- Third, we will clear away and wash away the stones, secretions and debris already formed, that hinder healing.

- Fourth, we will use herbs and special food factors to hasten healing, being very careful to use pure products

This will be done by a very powerful, parasite cleansing program and various other methods should the reader feel it's necessary for their respective condition. It goes into details that we do not have room to presently share. For this reason, we recommend the following book that entails the best parasite, kidney and liver cleansing program we know of and have personally used, see "The Cure For All Diseases," by Hulda Regehr Clark, Ph.D., N.D.

NEW DANGERS AND ALTERNATIVES OF FOOD & BEVERAGE INFORMATION

Coffee

According to How To Eat To live, the Messenger states that coffee is good to drink if done so in moderation. The intent of this book is not to debate on its pros and cons, but to point out certain factors to aid in making the coffee drinker aware of various aspects. The safest approach in making coffee is knowing how to prepare it. Percolating coffee or the drip method is two of the most unhealthiest ways, as opposed to the French Press and Vacuum methods. This is so largely due to the fact that with the percolator and dripping, as the water is heated up and filters over the coffee grounds, the amount of time it boils over 3 to 4 minutes, whether over the drip pot electric coils or through the percolator tube, a chemical called tannin is in the coffee bean but is not released so readily as from the fragile tea leaf. The longer coffee is boiled the more tannic acid is released.

Many different acidic constituents are present in coffee. Coffee's acids include malic acid, tannic acid, maleic acid, oleic acid, oxalic acid (which will be discussed further when discussing black and green teas), caffeic acid and chlorogenic acid, among others. These acidic constituents are responsible for the overall acidity of coffee and the discomfort that occasionally arises from the ingestion of this acidic beverage.

Furthermore, coffee contains caffeine, which, upon ingestion, causes the gastric secretion of acids. Accordingly, coffee drinking not only results in the ingestion of an acidic beverage, but also stimulates the production of additional acids.

Commonly, the coffee drinker's solution to discomfort arising from coffee's acidity is to either reduce the number of cups of coffee consumed each day (moderation as taught by Elijah Muhammad), avoid drinking coffee entirely, or alternatively, dilute the coffee, or accompany coffee drinking, with dairy products such as milk or cream. For the coffee drinker who eats one meal a day and has that meal in the evening, cream in that coffee coats the empty stomach from acid. There is a myth that black coffee is superior for some reason, but it is very hard on the lining of an empty stomach that has no protection from the early morning acids. Unfortunately, the use of dairy products as a solution to the problem of coffee acidity is not universal. Many people, including some coffee drinkers, suffer from lactose intolerance and have difficulty in digesting milk sugars. For these individuals, the problem of coffee acidity is not solved by the addition of milk products to coffee. Lastly, the acid can be reduced to a minimum by not boiling the coffee at all, this is done by using a Vacuum Pot or French Press.

Tea

Tea is used by more than one-half the human race; and, although the United States is not a tea-drinking country, one and one-half pounds are consumed per capita per annum.

All tea is grown from one species of shrub. Both green tea and black tea come from the leaves of the plant Camellia sinensis, however the processing that the leaves undergo to make the final tea is different. The leaves for black tea are fully oxidized while those for green teas are lightly steamed before being dried. The leaves of which constitute the tea of commerce. Climate, elevation, soil, cultivation, and care in picking and curing all go to make up the differences. First-quality tea is made from young, whole leaves. Two kinds of tea are considered: Black tea, made from leaves which have been allowed to ferment before curing. Green tea, made from unfermented leaves artificially colored.

The stimulating property of tea is due to the alkaloid, theine, together with an essential oil; it contains an astringent, tannin. Black tea contains less theine, essential oil, and tannin than green tea. The tannic acid, developed from the tannin by infusion, injures the coating of the stomach.

Although tea is not a substitute for food, it appears so for a considerable period of time, as its stimulating effect is immediate.

Tea should always be infused, never boiled. Long steeping destroys the delicate flavor by developing a larger amount of tannic acid.

Tea also contains oxalic acid and it is said to be conducive to kidney stone formation.
Oxalic acid crystals are as sharp as broken glass. All lower back pain can be cured by removing the sharp crystals in the kidneys. Our bodies make eight or more different kinds of kidney "stones." The oxalic acid variety is associated with sharp stabbing pains. In its effort to eliminate this extremely vicious acid your body neutralizes it with calcium first to make calcium oxalate. Your kidneys can keep a bit of calcium oxalate in solution but not a lot. The excess hardens into crystals. A glass of regular or iced tea (not herb tea or green tea) has about 20 mg8 of oxalic acid – way too much for kidneys to excrete. Tea is a toxic drink, not to be considered a beverage. Chocolate is very high in oxalate, too, and should not be used as a beverage (as cocoa). Children should never drink tea or cocoa. Their delicate kidneys should not be faced with the daily burden of excreting large amounts of oxalic acid. And calcium used to neutralize oxalic acid is wasted.

Calcium is a precious nutrient. It should be conserved for children's bone development.

Milk

In the Messenger's books he prescribes that we drink whole milk, which is clear of TB germs and that this is best for us; however, if we are subjected to the general dairies, we should boil it at a certain temperature to kill that germ. There are also other aspects associated with today's dairy milk we want to include in your preventive measures.
Pasteurization exposes (a food, as milk, cheese or yogurt) to an elevated temperature for a period of time sufficient to destroy certain microorganisms, as those that can produce disease or cause spoilage or undesirable fermentation of food, without radically altering taste or quality. This process also destroys many, if not, most of the nutrients in the milk, but more dangerous than that is the process of homogenization.

The homogenization process in either milk or cheese is unnatural. When you consume a dairy product that has been homogenized, it will cause the arteries to get scarred. These are the three major causes of arteriosclerosis. Arteriosclerosis is a degenerative change in the arteries, characterized by thickening of the vessel walls and accumulation of calcium with consequent loss of elasticity and lessened blood flow.

Cheese

Rennet and Coagulating Enzymes

What are coagulating enzymes and how do they create cheese?

According to Whole Food Market, "In order for milk to coagulate and eventually become cheese, enzymes must be added to breakdown the proteins that keep milk a liquid. Some enzymes do this better than others, but all of these enzymes are in the protein breaking subclass known as proteases. The best proteases or coagulants for making cheese are the type that break a specific protein called kappa casein. When the kappa casein is broken the milk loses its liquid infrastructure and begins to coagulate.

What are Rennet, Rennin, and Chymosin?

Rennet is defined in Webster's Unabridged Dictionary as "the lining membrane of the fourth stomach of the calf (and/or) a preparation or extract of the rennet membrane, used to curdle milk, as in making cheese...." Rennet is also used broadly to describe any enzyme used for the coagulation of milk in the process of making cheese.
Rennin is defined as "a coagulating enzyme occurring in the gastric juice of the calf, forming the active principal of rennet and able to curdle

milk." The cheese industry uses a broader definition of the term rennin, referring to it as "any enzyme used for the controlled coagulation of milk."
Chymosin, often used as another word for rennin, is the most common enzyme recovered from rennet.

Types Of Coagulating Enzymes Used To Make Cheese

Animal rennin is the coagulating enzyme (rennin or chymosin) that is harvested from the stomachs of calves.

Vegetable rennet is a misnomer given that the definition of rennet recognizes it strictly as an animal derived substance. Although cheese has been made using enzymes from the Lady Bedstraw, Stinging Nettle, and Thistle flower, the term vegetable rennet is most commonly used when describing enzymes produced using microbes. "Vegetable rennet" is sometimes used more generally to describe any non-animal rennet.

Microbial rennets are enzymes derived from a controlled fermentation of a fungus (e.g., Mucor Pusillus, Mucor Miehi, and Endothia Cryphonectria) or microbial rennets. However, microbial rennets cannot be used to produce cheddar or hard cheeses, limiting their application as an alternative to animal or bioengineered rennets.

Genetically engineered rennets. Shortages and fluctuations in the available supplies of calf rennet prompted the development of genetically engineered rennet. Food scientists can however produce a continuous and pure source of microbial chymosin by incorporating a calf's prochymosin gene into a microorganism. The first microbial chymosin was affirmed GRAS (generally recognized as safe) by the FDA in 1989, with many others following shortly thereafter. Currently, it is estimated that 50% of the chymosin used is produced by transgenic means.

Rennetless. The term "rennetless" is used to mean two things in the cheese world. First, rennetless cheeses are also called "acid precipitated cheeses" and include cottage cheese, ricotta, and some mozzarella. These types of cheese are created using their natural acid levels and do not require the addition of a coagulating enzyme. The second interpretation of "rennetless" cheese is any cheese made without the use of animal derived coagulants.

Why Is Rennet Controversial?

Historically rennet was extracted from calf stomachs by killing the calves, cutting the stomach into strips, scraping the lining to remove surface fat, stretching it onto racks where moisture is removed, grinding it and then finally mixing it with a salt solution until the rennin is extracted. Today the use of animal rennin is controversial to a variety of cheese consumers. The main positions are subdivided below.

Animal rights. Animal rights activists argue that it is inhumane to kill calves for their stomach enzymes, especially when there are several alternative coagulants available to make cheese. These activists would argue that if you eat cheese, then purchase one that is made using cloned or microbial enzymes.

Vegetarianism. Vegetarians can have a confusing time trying to figure out what type of coagulant is acceptable in their cheese. While some vegetarians would strictly adhere to a non-dairy diet, others who eat dairy are content to allow microbial coagulants and some can accept cloned chymosin as a reasonable alternative to using calf rennet. Several vegetarian organizations accept the use of cloned animal enzymes as a reasonable alternative to the animal rennet derived from the killing of calves.

Bioengineering. Genetic engineering has brought new ways to create chymosin for use in cheese making. Originally, a prochymosin gene was injected into a host strain of E Coli K-12, creating a tiny enzyme factory that produced an extremely pure and recoverable chymosin for use in cheese production. Current technology cuts genes from a calf cell and injects it into the genomes of bacteria and yeast. This produces high quality chymosin that is not subject to the volatile market for animal derived rennet. It is estimated that 70% of domestic cheese is produced with bioengineered chymosin. For a consumer who does not want bioengineered foods, animal or microbial rennet should be their choice.

Religion. Some orthodox religions (Jewish and Islam) have specific requirements and prohibitions for the consumption of meat products that can preclude the use of animal rennet. For example, information received from Dr. Chaudry of the Islamic Food and Nutrition Council of America (IFNCA), stated that for a food to be "Halal" (permitted for consumption by Muslims), it must be void of certain animal products and processing procedures. In this case, cheeses that are made from animal rennet are only excluded if the calf is slaughtered improperly or is contaminated with other prohibited ingredients or procedures. The IFNCA recommends the use of microbial or bioengineered chymosin for cheese making.

Current Problems With Cheese Coagulants

There are two major problems that arise for consumers and buyers when trying to distinguish the types of rennet in a particular cheese.

Labeling. There is no requirement for a cheese ingredient label to distinguish between the types of rennet that it may or may not contain. In fact, a cursory review of cheese labels at our 6th and Lamar store in Austin, Texas revealed at least 8 different ways that the coagulating enzymes were identified. They include, *enzymes, microbial enzymes, microbial enzymes* (non-animal, rennetless), *rennetless, rennet, enzymes and rennet, vegetarian rennet,* and *microbial coagulants.* A significant portion of the surveyed cheese labels simply said *enzymes*, while several labels did not list the type of coagulant used at all.

Obviously this type of labeling hurts cheese buyers as well as consumers. For a store cheese buyer, it is a challenge to track down cheeses that list the type(s) of coagulants used, while for the consumer, buying cheese products with a full understanding of the ingredients is next to impossible. Some companies have taken the time to list whether the cheese they make contains a particular type of enzyme, but these are few and far between.

Enzyme mixing. Compounding the labeling problem is the fact that cheese producers can mix animal, plant, and microbial enzymes under one ingredient listing called "enzymes". The FDA determined that it would be impractical for individual cheese packers to have on hand all the variations of labels needed to properly designate all cheese enzyme mixtures."

Last word, the Honorable Muhammad stated in How to Eat to Live, that we shouldn't eat a lot of aged cheese and that cream cheese is easier to digest.

ALTERNATIVES: Your own cow, your own farm, or pure organic without the processes associated.

Water

No matter what they are called, there are in fact more toxic chemicals in our water and food supply than ever before in history. These poisons are getting into our bodies primarily by:

- Drinking the water
- Eating or drinking anything made with water
- Eating any food that was grown with the water
- Eating any meat, poultry, fish, or dairy where the animal drank water
- Showering, bathing or swimming in water
- How toxins get in your body through your skin

The skin is the largest organ in the body. Anything put on the skin is absorbed and gets into the body. Even science admits this to be true. Since our skin is the largest organ in the body, it has been reported that we absorb more toxins by taking one shower than by drinking five glasses of water. In a shower, not only is the water with all the toxins being absorbed through the skin, many of the most volatile and dangerous toxins are turned into a gas created by the steam. These toxic fumes in your shower are then inhaled. A shower is practically a gas chamber filled with poisonous gas chemicals. Steam rooms, hot tubs and swimming pools are places where you will absorb the highest levels of toxins. The paradox is we think of these particular areas as being the healthiest.

The poisoned water supply is another significant factor relating to how toxins get into our body. By now it won't surprise you to learn how we are being misled by the news media and government agencies about the purity and safety of our water supply. Remember that chlorine and fluoride are the two main poisons that are in our water supply and are the reason our water is so unhealthy. Yet, the government and news media rates the quality of our water based on the amount of chlorine and fluoride in it! The more chlorine and fluoride in the water the healthier it is, claims the government! They even say that tap water is better than spring water because tap water has chlorine and fluoride in it and spring water does not. This is yet another way you are being lied to, deceived and brainwashed into thinking that chemicals are better than something in a natural state.

What about carbonated sodas?

The Messenger said that no intelligent person would drink them. One reason is because of the chemical sweeteners; whereas, they are some of the most toxic things you could put in your body. The problem, however, with virtually all carbonated beverages is they block calcium absorption. Calcium is one of the most important building blocks of nutrition.

According to the National Soft Drink Association (NSDA), consumption of soft drinks is now over 600 12-ounce servings (12 oz.) per person per year. Since 1978, soda consumption in the us has tripled for boys and doubled for girls. Young males age 12-29 are the biggest consumers at over 160 gallons per year-that's almost 2 quarts per day. At these levels, the calories from soft drinks contribute as much as 10 percent of the total daily caloric intake for a growing boy.

TARGETING THE YOUNG

Huge increases in soft drink consumption have not happened by chance-they are due to intense marketing efforts by soft drink corporations. Coca Cola, for example, has set the goal of raising consumption of its products in the US by at least 25 percent per year. The adult market is stagnant so kids are the target.

According to an article in Beverage, January 1999, "Influencing elementary school students is very important to soft drink marketers." Since the 1960s the industry has increased the single-serving size from a standard 6-½-ounce bottle to a 20- ounce bottle. At movie theaters and at 7-Eleven stores the most popular size is now the 64-ounce "Double Gulp."

Soft drink companies spend billions on advertising. Much of these marketing efforts are aimed at children through playgrounds, toys, cartoons, movies, videos, charities and amusement parks; and through contests, sweepstakes, games and clubs via television, radio, magazines and the internet. Their efforts have paid off. Last year soft drink companies grossed over $57 billion in sales in the us alone, a colossal amount.

In 1998 the Center for Science in the Public Interest (CSPI) warned the public that soft drink companies were beginning to infiltrate our schools and kid clubs. For example, they reported that Coca-Cola paid the Boys & Girls Clubs of America $60 million to market its brand exclusively in over 2000 facilities. Fast food companies selling soft drinks now run ads on Channel One, the commercial television network with programming shown in classrooms almost every day to eight million middle, junior and high school students. In 1993, District 11 in Colorado Springs became the first public school district in the us to place ads for Burger King in its hallways and on the sides of its school buses. Later, the school district signed a 10-year deal with Coca-Cola, bringing in $11 million during the life of the contract. This arrangement was later imitated all over Colorado. The contracts specify annual sales quotas with the result that school administrators encourage students to drink sodas, even in the classrooms. One high school in Beltsville, Maryland, made nearly $100,000 last year on a deal with a soft drink company.

While our children are exposed to unremitting publicity for soft drinks, evidence of their dangers accumulates. The consumption of soft drinks, like land-mine terrain, is riddled with hazards. We as practitioners and advocates of a healthy life-style recognize that consuming even as little as one or two sodas per day is undeniably connected to a myriad of pathologies. The most commonly associated health risks are obesity, diabetes and other blood sugar disorders, tooth decay, osteoporosis and bone fractures, nutritional deficiencies, heart disease, food addictions and eating disorders, neurotransmitter dysfunction from chemical sweeteners, and neurological and adrenal disorders from excessive caffeine.

EARLY WARNINGS

Warnings about the dangers of soft drink consumption came to us as early as 1942 when the American Medical Association's (AMA) Council on Food and Nutrition made the following noble statement:

"From the health point of view it is desirable especially to have restriction of such use of sugar as is represented by consumption of sweetened carbonated beverages and forms of candy which are of low nutritional value. The Council believes it would be in the interest of the public health for all practical means to be taken to limit consumption of sugar in any form in which it fails to be combined with significant proportions of other foods of high nutritive quality."

Since that time the first notable public outcry came in 1998, 56 years later, when the CSPI published a paper called "Liquid Candy" blasting the food industry for "mounting predatory marketing campaigns [especially] aimed at children and adolescents." At a press conference, CSPI set up 868 cans of soda to represent the amount of soda the average young male consumed during the prior year. For additional shock effect, CSPI displayed baby bottles with soft drink logos such as Pepsi, Seven-up and Dr. Pepper, highlighting a study that "found that parents are four times more likely to feed their children soda pop when their children use those logo bottles than when they don't." In "Liquid Candy" CSPI revealed that even though, over a period of fifty years, soft drink production increased nine times and by 1998 ".provided more than one-third of all refined sugars in the diet, . . . the AMA and other health organizations [remained] largely silent."

How could the medical community and we as responsible citizens concerned with health policy have been apathetic for a half a century? Considering this question makes me feel like a tired old guard dog that knows he is ignoring his responsibilities, but is too worn down to do anything about them. Even if inertia were not a problem, the money and effort required to launch a public interest campaign to stand up to the soft drink industry would be Herculean if not impossible. In the meantime, the relentlessly ambitious and wealthy soft drink companies with their very hip life-style ads manage to seduce ever-increasing numbers of consumers, most of them our kids.

INGREDIENTS IN SOFT DRINKS-A WITCH'S BREW

High Fructose Corn Syrup, now used in preference to sugar, is associated with poor development of collagen in growing animals, especially in the context of copper deficiency. All fructose must be metabolized by the liver. Animals on high-fructose diets develop liver problems similar to those of alcoholics.

Aspartame, used in diet sodas, is a potent neurotoxin and endocrine disrupter.

Caffeine stimulates the adrenal gland without providing nourishment. In large amounts, caffeine can lead to adrenal exhaustion, especially in children.

Phosphoric acid, added to give soft drinks "bite," is associated with calcium loss.

Citric acid often contains traces of MSG, a neurotoxin.

Artificial Flavors may also contain traces of MSG.

Water may contain high amounts of **fluoride** and other contaminants.

GI DISTRESS

One common problem seen over the years, especially in teenagers, is general gastrointestinal (GI) distress. This includes increased stomach acid levels requiring acid inhibitors and moderate to severe gastric inflammation with possible stomach lining erosion. The common complaint I hear is chronic "stomach ache." In almost every case, when the client successfully abstains from sodas and caffeine, the symptoms will go away.

What causes these symptoms? We know that many soda brands contain caffeine and that caffeine does increase stomach acid levels. What we may not be aware of is that sodas also contain an array of chemical acids as additives, such as acetic, fumaric, gluconic and phosphoric acids, all of them synthetically produced. That is why certain sodas work so well when used to clean car engines. For human consumption, however, the effects are much less satisfying and quite precarious. Drinking sodas, especially on an empty stomach, can upset the fragile acid-alkaline balance of the stomach and other gastric lining, creating a continuous acid environment. This prolonged acid environment can lead to inflammation of the stomach and duodenal lining which becomes quite painful. Over the long term, it can lead to gastric lining erosion.

Another problem with sodas is that they act as dehydrating diuretics, much like tea, coffee and alcohol. All of these drinks can inhibit proper digestive function. It is much healthier to consume herbal teas, nutritional soups and broths, naturally lacto-fermented beverages and water to supply our daily fluid needs. These fluids support, not inhibit, digestion.

SPORTS DRINKS

Students are now being given "electrolyte" drinks called "ergogenic aids" to replace electrolytes that are allegedly depleted during workouts. There are three problems with using these drinks as a rehydration solution. First, most soft drinks are diuretics, meaning they squeeze liquids out of the body, thus exacerbating dehydration instead of correcting it. Second, most people actually lose few electrolytes during exercise. After exercise the body is usually in an electrolyte load having lost more fluids than electrolytes.

If sweating has been profuse, electrolytes can be replaced by drinking a lacto-fermented beverage or pure mineral water, which contains a proper ratio of minerals (electrolytes), and by eating a healthy diet containing Celtic sea salt. Third, when we give sugar-laden drinks to dehydrated kids, the high sugar content requires that blood be sent to the stomach to digest it. This fluid shift can lower the blood volume in other parts of the body making them more susceptible to cramps and heat-related illnesses.

STIMULANT SOFT DRINKS AND VIOLENCE

The industry has begun to market so-called stimulant soft drinks, which usually consist of higher-than-usual levels of caffeine, along with other compound stimulants. According to an article published in The Lancet, December 2000, the Irish government ordered "urgent research" into the effects of so-called "functional energy" or stimulant soft drinks after the death of an 18-year-old who died while playing basketball. He had consumed three cans of "Red Bull," a stimulant soft drink. The article noted there have been reports of a rise in aggressive late-night violence occurring when people switch to these drinks while drowsy from too much alcohol. The resulting violence was so pervasive that some establishments in Ireland have refused to sell stimulant drinks. The entire European community has taken the problem seriously enough to ask the EU's scientific community to examine stimulant sodas and their effect on food and health safety, but no such outcry has been heard in the us.

BONE FRACTURES

Over the last 30 years a virtual tome of information has been published linking soft drink consumption to a rise in osteoporosis and bone fractures. New evidence has shown an alarming rise in deficiencies of calcium and other minerals and resulting bone fractures in young girls. A 1994 report published in the Journal of Adolescent Health summarizes a small study (76 girls and 51 boys) and points toward an increasing and "strong association between cola beverage consumption and bone fractures in girls." High calcium intake offered some protection. For boys, only low total caloric intake was associated with a higher risk of bone fractures. The study concluded with the following: "The high consumption of carbonated beverages and the declining consumption of milk are of great public health significance for girls and women because of their proneness to osteoporosis in later life."

A larger, cross sectional retrospective study of 460 high school girls was published in Pediatrics & Adolescent Medicine in June 2000. The study indicated that cola beverages were "highly associated with bone fractures." In their conclusion the authors warned that, ". . . national concern and alarm about the health impact of carbonated beverage consumption on teenaged girls is supported by the findings of this study".

THE BATTLE AHEAD

The dangers of society's other drinking problem have recently been in the news. Senator Christopher Dodd and Representative George Miller have commissioned a study on the uses and oversight of school vending machines. Pending legislation in the State of Maryland would turn school soda vending machines off during the school day. Senator Patrick Leahy has introduced a bill requiring the usDA to rule within 18 months on banning or limiting the sale of soda and junk food in schools before students have eaten lunch.

The soft drink industry has fought back by funding four studies on soft drink consumption at the Georgetown Center for Food and Nutrition Policy. Predictably, these studies found that there was nothing wrong with soft drinks. In fact, researchers said they found a positive relationship between soft drink consumption and exercise. All this means is that those children participating in sports programs drank more sodas.

The National Association of Secondary School Principals (NAASP) says that decisions about soda sales should be made at the local level and not by the federal government. School administrators are caught between demands of a few parents for a saner food policy and the need for more funds in the face of dwindling school budgets.

One good idea comes from the Philippines, a country where malnutrition is an ominous health threat. A recently devised plan there would allow citizens to cash in on the country's "junk food diet" by taxing every liter bottle of carbonated soft drink sold. If the us taxed soft drink sales, the new income stream generated could then be distributed to declining school budgets. Is this not a better idea than forcing our schools to sell their souls to soft drink companies under the titanic sink of fiscal degradation?

The alarm has been sounded! Are you listening? I strongly encourage all who are concerned about the health of their families to consider the debilitating consequences of drinking soft drinks. How many more studies and reports need to be published before we notice the tsunami lurking ahead? In the 1970s, we finally recognized the risks of smoking. In the 1990s, the problem of teenage drinking became widely known. The new millennium is the time for awakening to the risks of soda consumption-America's other drinking problem.

Phosphoric Acid and Tooth Rot

Now that soft drinks are sold in almost all public and private schools, dentists are noticing a condition in teenagers that used to be found only in the elderly-a complete loss of enamel on the teeth, resulting in yellow teeth. The culprit is phosphoric acid in soft drinks, which causes tooth rot as well as digestive problems and bone loss. Dentists are reporting complete loss of the enamel on the front teeth in teenaged boys and girls who habitually drink sodas.

Normally the saliva is slightly alkaline, with a pH of about 7.4. When sodas are sipped throughout the day, as is often the case with teenagers, the phosphoric acid lowers the pH of the saliva to acidic levels. In order to buffer this acidic saliva, and bring the pH level above 7 again, the body pulls calcium ions from the teeth. The result is a very rapid depletion of the enamel coating on the teeth. When dentists do cosmetic bonding, they first roughen up the enamel with a chemical compound-that chemical is phosphoric acid! Young people who must have all their yellowed front teeth cosmetically bonded have already done part of the dentist's job, by roughening up the tooth surface with phosphoric acid.

Recently the National Institutes of Health held a conference on dental decay worldwide. The speakers discussed many possible causes and solutions, but not one mentioned the known effects of phosphoric acid in soft drinks!

Fruit Juices

Consumers often drink commercial fruit juices in the belief that they are healthier than soft drinks. However, the manufacture of fruit juices is a highly industrialized process. Orange juice, for example, is made in huge quantities. The entire orange is squeezed and goes into the tank, which means that neurotoxic cholinesterase inhibitor pesticide sprays on the peel end up in the juice. Although the juice is pasteurized under high temperatures and pressures, pressure-resistent and temperature-resistant fungi and molds can remain in the juice. Many mutagenic factors have been detected in commercial orange juice. A compound made of soy protein and pectin is added to orange juice so that it remains opaque and doesn't settle.

Other fruits, such as grapes, present additional problems because of the large amounts of fluoride-containing pesticides used on the crops. Fruit juices are very high in sugar and have actually been more detrimental to the teeth of test animals than sodas!

If you want to drink fruit juice, buy a juicer and make your own with organic fruit.

Juices

What about juices? The Messenger does say raw juice is better, but says as well that we should not drink too much raw juices. He points out that the insects have feed on them. Another aspect of this precaution is that, if you've ever gone to see how these products are made, you would see why. People think juice is juice is juice. It's simply not true! Walking out in your yard and picking your own, peeling it and juicing would produce you a good glass of organic juice. Well how is that different from juice you buy at the store? A couple of major differences:

Remember, it's all about the money. The people who sell these products are trying to sell more products at a lower cost. How do they do that? Well, first and foremost let's take orange juice. What will happen is they'll find the worst oranges in the world that they couldn't sell, and that's what they make their juice from. Keep in mind that these oranges have been produced in the "conventional" ways, with chemical fertilizers, pesticides, herbicides and genetic engineering. That is what’s meant by conventional.

They then pick the fruit that can't be sold, and that's what they make the juice from. The problem is that in the processing of the juice in the plants, bacteria and mold can easily develop, contaminating the product. So by law the product has to be pasteurized, which means the product has to be heated to 220 degrees for thirty minutes to kill any amount of bacteria so you don't get sick as you drink it. This kills all the living natural enzymes and destroys the natural energy surrounding that natural fruit. It is then filtered, and in many cases sugar, which is not listed on the label, is added to make the product sweeter. If sugar is not added, the filtering process and the pasteurization process make the product much sweeter. So you are getting a product that is much, much sweeter than in nature. The best example of this is filtered apple juice. When you look at apple juice that is super clear, it has no living enzymes, and it's virtually a massive sugar high. It's just a man made product under the disguise of a natural, healthy product. It's not healthy; it's man made, it's tainted with chemicals and toxins, and because of the processing is just not healthy. Juice is good, but only if you make it in your home with organic fruits, and drink your juice right away, and even then, as before mentioned, with moderation. Once you have juiced the product and air gets to it, it begins to oxidize and lose its nutritional value; therefore, if you have a juice machine in your house, you get organic fruits, you make juice and you drink it.

Messenger Elijah Muhammad prescribes that fruit be eaten raw. So, why should you drink juice anyway? That's a very, very good question. 100 years ago we didn't have juice machines. The answer is this: Even if you buy organic fruits and vegetables today, because over the years the soil has been depleted of much of its nutritional value and energy, today's fruits and vegetables don't have the energy or the nutritional value that they did 100 years ago. Even organic fruits and vegetables have less than they did 100 years ago. So a good alternative is to juice them. The nutritional value and the life force energy is in the juice. The fiber in the fruits is still needed for other bodily functions such as the elimination through the colon, so you still need to eat the whole fruit and vegetable. But you can get the nutritional value through the juice. Messenger Elijah Muhammad prescribes eating certain vegetables raw, while most he prescribes to be eaten cooked, preferably steamed. Consult books 1 & 2 of How To Eat To Live for details. It is much better than taking vitamin and mineral tablets if you're going to juice.

BEEF, PORK, POULTRY & FISH

Beef & Mad Cow Disease

In How To Eat To Live, Messenger Elijah Muhammad points out specifically and clearly that no meat is good for you, because it is too hard for humans to digest. He goes on to say that "If you must eat meat," eat lamb, because of its better digestive properties. Although he teaches that beef is more coarser than lamb, it is safer to eat than pork.

Over the years, the means by which farmers have commercialized on cattle and other livestock has made them resort to worse methods of feeding them. This is a better reason to stop eating meat than it simply being too coarse for your digestives system.

For decades British and North American farmers have been feeding their beef and dairy cattle, which are of course herbivores, cheap protein supplements made from things, which include sheep brains, spinal cords, and other animal parts. Sheep, as any farmer will testify, have for centuries carried scrapie--a fatal, degenerative brain disease, which is remarkably similar to Mad Cow Disease and CJD. It is feared that this disease can be transmitted to humans who eat meat from infected cattle.

Since 1989 Britain has banned sheep offal (the ground remains of the dead animal) from cattle feed. Indeed, all mammal tissue has been banned from all agricultural feed in that country, and, furthermore, the World Health Organization is now endorsing a ban for all countries.

However, in the United States this practice continues up to the present time as a routine process, designed to boost milk and meat production. Indeed, offal from sheep, cattle and other animals, as well as animal feces, is routinely fed to American food animals (cattle, pigs, poultry and fish) in the form of rendered pellets, powder or meal. In addition, massive quantities of blood meal, bone meal and other animal byproducts find their way into food animal's feed. It is grossly unnatural and dangerous to feed blood and other animal parts to cattle, which are natural vegetarians. Animal diseases may very well be passed on in the process.
Various diseases may also be transmitted to human beings who eat infected animals. Indeed, from feed, to cow, to the human brain, appears to be the progression of Mad Cow Disease, which has leaped across the species barrier to become a varian of CJD.

Cattle with the disease show symptoms of staggering, drooling, aggression, and confused behavior, appearing to have gone "mad." Afflicted humans show symptoms similar to Alzheimer's disease--dementia, confusion, convulsions, loss of speech, sight, and hearing, and ending with a coma and death. This disease, one of the most mysterious known to human beings, is always fatal and there is no treatment for it. The incubation period seems to be four to thirty years.

The causative agent appears to be a deformed molecule called a "prion," (pronounced PREE-on), a mysterious and abnormal infectious protein. This strange-acting, never-before-seen infectious agent, which is neither a bacteria nor a virus, is distinct from anything encountered before--an infectious agent that defies the accepted rules of nature. Smaller than the tiniest virus, they do not contain nucleic acid which makes up the RNA and DNA that carry the genetic codes of normal viruses, bacteria, plants, cows, humans and virtually all other living things. Yet they are able to replicate and spread, but do not activate an immune response. Unfortunately, they are highly resistant to heat, UV light, radiation and most common chemical disinfectants.

Pork – The Other White Meat

New Image, Same Flesh

"Underway is an "on-farm program" to certify pigs as free ["Free" is defined based on good farm management] of trichina parasites. Attempts are feverishly being made that could become a model for excluding other meat borne diseases from foods.
The parasitic worm and the false illusion that makes U.S. consumers cook pork chops and roasts to the consistency of shoe leather may be getting a little help. Thinking that "properly cooking" the poison flesh will make it safe to eat has been one of the standard justification, or shall we say, rationalizations, for evading the facts against eating the flesh of swine.

"Thanks to changes in the way most producers and the government will be re-defining the term "free" when it comes to pork, sellers of this divinely prohibited flesh will possibly be able to one day see labels of the meat that says trichinae free. During the last decade, for example, the percentage of U.S. swine infected with Trichinella spiralis varied, depending on the population surveyer; yet, one thing was for sure, all eaters are infected in some degree.

As before stated, most human infections go undetected; consequently, "during the 1990s, fewer than 50 cases of human trichinellosis were reported each year to the Centers for Disease Control and Prevention, compared to 500 cases annually in the 1940s"

"Still, "pork suffers from its legacy and parasites," says Agricultural Research Service parasitologist H. Ray Gamble. The shadow of the worm not only keeps Americans overcooking fresh pork, it also closes many markets overseas.

"That's about to change. Starting this summer, an innovative program for certifying pork trichinae-free "based on good farm management" is going through its final shakedown--a 2-year pilot study. The national certification program is expected to be a model for controlling other food borne pathogens--including bacteria--at the source of infection, says Gamble. He heads the Parasite Biology and Epidemiology Laboratory in Beltsville, Maryland.

"Gamble is collaborating on the project with the National Pork Producers Council (NPPC), the meatpacking industry, and two other USDA agencies--the Animal and Plant Health Inspection Service (APHIS) and the Food Safety Inspection Service (FSIS).

How It Will Work

"The NPPC encourages pork producers to volunteer for certification by having their operations audited by an APHIS-accredited veterinarian. APHIS will train and qualify these vets to educate producers on "good management practices" (to satisfy the "free" definition) and to conduct the audits. Using a standardized checklist, the vets will be looking for practices that would prevent the herd's exposure to raw garbage, animal waster, etc.... On many farms, and as a recognized practice, pigs will eat infected carcasses or any other dead, whether infected or not. The production sites that pass muster (the defined parameters) will be certified as having safe management practices.

"Participating packing plants will keep certified pigs separate from uncertified pigs and follow a protocol developed with FSIS. FSIS will confirm that the pigs from certified sites are handled separately and will also oversee spot testing of the animals to ensure they are, in fact, trichinae free (the trichina parasites fall within a 0.3 minimum to a 1.0 maximum count per cubic flesh inch).
"It's a voluntary program--a first for FSIS," says John Ragan, national livestock program leader for FSIS' Animal Production Food Safety Program.

"Interest in such a program solidified around 1994. That's when an E. coli outbreak caused by tainted hamburgers from a fast-food restaurant heightened national interest in food safety, says Larry Miller, senior staff veterinarian with APHIS' Veterinary Services.

"Government and industry began to look for ways to improve safety at the farm level.

"We'll run the pilot study like a bona fide program, only on a small scale, to find the bugs and fix them," Miller says. "Then, we'll scale it up incrementally."

"Dave Pyburn, director of veterinary science at NPPC, expects certification to begin in earnest in 2001, when the pilot study is scheduled to end. "We've designed the program with the idea that 90 to 95 percent of pork-producing sites will volunteer for the audit," he says.
"Gamble says the meatpackers, who want to improve their product's image, have been a driving force in supporting the concept of on-farm certification. (since we can't totally remove the parasite, let us just work on the public relations and change the way it's viewed).

"Countries in the European Union (EU) test each pig carcass for the presence of trichinae worms--at a cost of $576 million in 1998. And they expect their trading partners to do the same. But carcass testing is too costly and cumbersome for U.S. packers, says Gamble. So the solution has been to strictly control the preparation of processed pork products, such as sausage and ham, and to re-educate the public to cook fresh pork thoroughly instead.

"The on-farm audit is an approach to food safety that holds promise of being superior to the individual testing of pigs at slaughter," says NPPC's Pyburn.

"As a member of the International Commission on Trichinellosis, Gamble has served as liaison between the on-farm certification program committee and the international community. But he doesn't expect EU countries to immediately start buying fresh U.S. pork certified under the proposed system. "Over time, when we have a track record of safety, these countries may accept on-farm certification," he says.

"Gamble also spearheaded a 2-year study of pork production farms in six northeastern states to validate the ELISA test and identify the management factors associated with trichinae-positive herds. Only 15 animals out of the 4,078 tested were positive. And those animals had too few worms to pose a public health risk, he says. However, the "health risk" is always defined a lot more loosely by the profit bearers. Additionally, the motivation to surpress the public fear of trichinellosis from pork plays itself out to a public relations campaign which aims to make the public believe that the actual threat is a perceive threat rather than a real one.

"Three years ago, Gamble and the other members of the Trichinae Working Group--a committee that oversees the certification efforts--enlisted a mid-western packing plant and pork producers in three states to test the feasibility of on-farm certification. The 6-month study did not find a single animal that tested positive (over recognized and acceptable levels) out of

220,000 pigs tested. Gamble adds that it validated the auditing system and demonstrated that the participating producers were already keeping their herds clear of potential exposure.

"He points out that research on the trichina parasite has a long history at the Beltsville (Maryland) Agricultural Research Center, so he began with plenty of information about the disease and its transmission. This knowledge made Trichinella the ideal organism for launching a whole new concept in food quality assurance." One such "new" concept, in an attempt to get around an old problem, is irradition.

WHAT IS IRRADIATION OF FOOD?

Food irradiation is a process by which food is exposed to a controlled source of ionizing radiation to prolong shelf life and reduce food losses, improve microbiologic safety, and/or reduce the use of chemical fumigants and additives. It can be used to reduce insect infestation of grain, dried spices, and dried or fresh fruits and vegetables; inhibit sprouting in tubers and bulbs; retard postharvest ripening of fruits; inactivate parasites in meats and fish; eliminate spoilage microbes from fresh fruits and vegetables; extend shelf life in poultry, meats, fish, and shellfish; decontaminate poultry and beef; and sterilize foods and feeds.

Irradiation kills microbes primarily by fragmenting DNA. The sensitivity of organisms increases with the complexity of the organism. Thus, viruses are most resistant to destruction by irradiation, and insects and parasites are most sensitive. Spores and cysts (what is lodged dormently in the swine's muscles waiting for human consumption) are quite resistant to the effects of irradiation, because they contain little DNA and are in highly stable resting states. Toxins and prions, which have few chemical bonds to disrupt, are resistant to irradiation. The conditions under which irradiation takes place (ie, temperature, humidity, and atmospheric content) can affect the dose required to achieve the food processing goal, but these are well-described and easily controlled.

American pork producers have always been aware of food borne illnesses. Food irradiation is a technology that holds promise in providing a safe and effective way to minimize the risk of food borne illnesses.

Food irradiation involves the use of ionizing energy to control bacteria or parasites in food. Notice the word "controlled" is used instead of eliminated. Irradiation has been approved for use by over 35 countries for more than 40 products. Irradiation has been endorsed by the United Nation's Food and Agriculture Organization (FAO) and the World Health Organization (WHO) as an important technology in reducing food losses due to insect pests, food spoilage and microbial contamination.

The Food and Drug Administration (FDA) regulates food irradiation as a food additive. FDA has approved irradiation for several food products. Pork is currently approved for processing at a low dose of 0.3 - 1.0 kiloGray (kGy) to inactivate (not eliminate) trichinae. Irradiated poultry and fruits have been distributed on a limited basis.

Because irradiation produces almost no heat within food, this makes many question the "properly cooked ploy." A recent check off funded study found that irradiation of pork had minimal to no effect on flavor, aroma, and textural attributes of chilled and frozen boneless pork chops. In addition, consumers found no difference between irradiated and control samples for overall acceptance, meatiness, freshness, tenderness, and juiciness.

In June 1994, Isomedix, Inc. submitted a petition to FDA to request approval for irradiation of fresh meat at levels up to 4.5 kGy and in frozen meat up to 7.0 kGy. On December 2, 1997, FDA granted approval for the irradiation of fresh and frozen beef, pork, and lamb. Approval of this petition will allow pork to be irradiated at medium doses, which would have a pasteurization effect and extend shelf life. However, before there is widespread adoption and use of irradiation technology, the U.S. Department of Agriculture must first write regulations on how irradiation is to be used and how products produced with this process are to be labeled. On February 24, 1999, USDA published the proposed rule to permit the use of ionizing radiation for treating fresh or frozen uncooked meat, pork and its byproducts, and certain meat food products to reduce levels of pathogens or parasites (control), not eliminate them.

There continues to be increased public interest in food safety issues and technologies to enhance safety. Consumer research has shown that the more consumers learn about irradiation, the more likely they are to accept irradiated products. Providing information on the process of irradiation and its benefits markedly influence consumer attitudes about purchasing irradiated products.

National Pork Producers Council continues to be supportive of food irradiation and strongly encourages USDA to expedite the finalization and expansion of the proposed rule for commercial plant usage of irradiation to all meat products. In extensive comments to the Agency, NPPC expressed concern about the limited scope of products covered by the FDA approval that will leave this proven technology unavailable for a number of products (e.g. raw and fully cooked, ready-to-eat, processed meat and poultry products) that could particularly benefit from this technology. In addition, USDA should take a leadership role in explaining the benefits of irradiation to the public and providing assurances about the safety of the process. NPPC believes that it would be appropriate to label pork as "fresh" if it is irradiated to levels approved by the FDA. [This does not imply that the pork will be completely absent of the parasite].

TRICHINAE HERD CERTIFICATION

(National Pork Producers Council)

"Trichinella spiralis, a nematode parasite, is found throughout the world and is capable of infecting many warm-blooded animals. Swine, fox, wolf, bear, rat, dog, cat, raccoon, skunk, opossum, and marine mammals are known reservoirs of Trichinella spiralis. Swine [inherently] infected [with]...Trichinella containing encysted larvae. Some of the most common [additional] modes of transmission to swine are:

"1. Feeding uncooked garbage containing meat or meat wrappers (organic waste products, manure, etc...)
2. Consumption of wildlife carcasses including rats, snakes when clearing swamps.
3. Cannibalism of infected swine carcasses (allowing hogs to eat their own young)

"The National Animal Health Monitoring System's National Swine Survey in 1995 showed a trichinae infection rate of 0.013%. Despite the fact that trichinosis is common in today's industry, U.S. pork is still stigmatized due to public perception and lack of education. The consumer's fear of trichinae causes them to either overcook or simply avoid eating pork. Trichinosis is also an impediment to reaching our full market potential internationally.

"NPPC in conjunction with several government agencies and allied industry launched the National Trichinae Research Project (NTRP) in 1994. The first portion of this project was the Northeast Trichinae Research Project in 1995-96. Pigs from 156 farms of various sizes and management types in New Jersey, Connecticut, Rhode Island, Massachusetts, Vermont, and New Hampshire were
included in the project.

"The on-farm risk factors for trichinae infection are: 1) feeding uncooked waste products, table scraps or animal carcasses to pigs; 2) exposure of pigs to live wildlife, including rodents; and 3) general farm hygiene practices and swine carcass removal and disposal methods.

"The second portion of this project was the Iowa Trichinae Certification Pilot Project in 1997. This project was broken down into two phases: 1) initial testing of all swine entering a northwest Iowa packing plant for a six month period to establish a trichinae prevalence for the farms marketing there; and 2) on-farm evaluation of trichinae infection risk factor analysis (an audit) and comparison with the in-plant testing results. Over 220,000 pigs were tested and all samples tested negative [or below levels we deemed safe and posed no public health risk] for trichinae. The audit contained questions concerning farm management, bio-security, feed and feed storage, rodent control programs, and general hygiene. In 1999-2000 the NTRP Working Group plans to implement the program in one or more large scale pilots that will closely emulate the final voluntary program. Several packing plants and production systems have contacted NPPC to volunteer to be a part of these large-scale pilots. These pilots will involve testing of all aspects of this proposed program from the farm to the retail counter to ensure delivery of known trichinae-safe pork. This is the last step in validating the on-farm certification process as a mechanism for producing trichinae-safe pork.

"If these projects are successful in developing and validating an on-farm certification system for trichinae-safe production practices, it will open the door to implementation of a system which will have a major impact on how U.S. fresh pork is viewed internationally and by our own consumers.

"Success is very likely due to several factors. The prevalence of swine trichinellosis is [acceptable at] low [levels] and the few remaining infected areas are easily identifiable. Farm management strategies for eliminating the [inherent] risk of infection are simple and usually easily implemented. Most management systems now in use lack trichinae infection risk factors and this can easily be documented and monitored through the certification process.

"...It was resolved that the United States pork industry should take aggressive steps to certify that U.S. pork products are trichinae free [as defined by the terms of the pork certification program] and communicate this information to the domestic and international pork chain.

"Trichinae certification is an approach to food safety that holds promise to being superior to individual testing of pigs at slaughter, which is the trichinae inspection process currently being used by countries we compete with in the international marketplace. Certification will allow the U.S. to better compete in the fresh pork international market and it will help to change the perceptions of pork our own domestic consumers hold. With this new technology and with the cooperation of producers, veterinarians, packers, and the government, we will be able to remove [change the perspective of] trichinae as a consumer concern.

Consuming Irradiated Food Has Not Been Shown To Be Safe

"On July 22, 1985, FDA announced that it had decided to allow the irradiation of fresh or previously frozen pork products to control the Trichinella spiralis parasite, the bug that causes trichinosis. This action came in response to an industry petition that had been filed one year earlier. The decision on retail labeling, however, was in the hands of the U.S. Department of Agriculture (USDA). Although USDA has said that labeling decisions would be made on a case by case basis, it has indicated that at the present time they will require that the labels include the word "irradiated" rather than the FDA's misleading term 'picowaved.'"

"Despite the green light given to food irradiation by the FDA, the Public Citizen Health Research Group has serious reservations about the safety of consuming irradiated foods. This concern is not allayed by the FDA approval since that approval was not based on animal studies designed to assess risk but rather was based on a calculation of the amount of chemical changes induced in the food by the irradiation process.

"When the FDA announced its proposal to allow irradiation of fruits and vegetables, it described the review of the safety of irradiation conducted by an internal agency task force, the Bureau of Foods' Irradiated Foods Committee (BFIC). This committee determined that the safety of irradiated food exposed to 100 krads of radiation or less could be presumed based on the "low level of total URPs" that would be created at such doses. URPs, or unique radiolytic products, are "new chemical constituents in the food...generated by the irradiation process." The same rationale was used in approving irradiation of pork. Thus, the BFIC, and FDA subsequently, did not rely on any tests of toxicity or carcinogenesis conducted in animals to conclude that irradiated food was safe for human consumption.

"Perhaps the main reason FDA did not rely on long term animal tests to assess the safety of irradiated food is that very few such tests exist. In addition, the animal tests that have been done were largely rejected by FDA as providing an inadequate basis for making a determination. An internal FDA review of 413 studies on the toxicity of irradiated foods found that 344 (84 percent) were either inconclusive or inadequate to demonstrate eitha safety or toxicity. Of the remaining studies, 32 indicated adverse effects and 37 appeared to support safety. The FDA memo states that "on detailed examination of these 69 studies [only] five studies (one percent of all studies reviewed) appeared to support safety."

"One recent set of studies that was not included in this review was carried out under the auspices of the USDA. This study, which was actually 12 different studies, examined the effect of feeding irradiated chicken to several animal species. One of these 12 studies found that fruit flies fed irradiated chicken had a statistically significant dose related increase in the rate of death of their offspring compared with flies who were not fed irradiated chicken.

In another of these studies, a long term study involving mice, the researchers found that mice fed irradiated chicken had a greater incidence of kidney disease than mice fed unirradiated chicken. In reviewing these findings, the group that did the work, Ralston Purina, concluded that "While no single finding from the study is highly illuminating, a collective assessment of study results argues against a definitive conclusion that the gamma irradiated test material was free of toxic properties."

"The results on kidney damage are consistent with another study in which kidney damage was found in rats fed irradiated food. In that study the authors stated that, “the severity of these changes was directly dependent on the dose of irradiation of the food products."

"Another study found testicular damage in rats fed irradiated food. Studies in both malnourished children and monkeys have demonstrated that consumption of freshly irradiated wheat may lead to an increase in abnormal white blood cells, a condition known as polyploidy.

"Other studies have found that animals fed irradiated food are more likely to experience chromosomal damage. After reviewing these and other studies on this issue, Dr. Jonathan Ward, an expert in genetic toxicology at the University of Texas, made the following statement in a letter to FDA Commissioner Young:

"These studies as a group fail to either prove or disprove the existence of a hazard from the use of irradiated food. It appears possible that unstable mutagenic products may be produced in foods by irradiation. It is difficult to believe that adequate tests of the effects of radiation on food can be conducted without individually evaluating the components of the foods for which radiation sterilization is intended."

WHAT IS THE CURRENT STATUS OF FOOD IRRADIATION IN THE UNITED STATES?

In 1991, Food Technology Services Incorporated opened the first dedicated food irradiation facility in North America near Tampa, Florida. Strawberries, tomatoes, and citrus fruit from this facility have been marketed directly to consumers in Florida and Illinois since 1992. Fruits from Hawaii, including papaya and lychees, were irradiated and sold in several states during 1995. Although irradiated spices and herbs have been approved for use since 1963, they have only been marketed in the United States since 1995. Vidalia onions irradiated in Florida have been marketed at the retail level in Chicago since 1992. Since 1993, small quantities of irradiated chicken have been available in retail outlets in Florida, Illinois, Iowa, and Kansas.

About 40 large-scale gamma facilities are in operation in the United States for sterilization of medical, surgical, and pharmaceutical products and packaging materials. In addition, 4 dedicated food irradiation facilities are currently in operation. Table 1 shows which foods are approved for irradiation in the United States market.

TABLE 1.

Rules From US FDA for Food Irradiation (*)

Food	Purpose of Irradiation
Spices, dry vegetable Seasoning	Decontamination/disinfest insects
Wheat, wheat powder	Disinfest insects
White potatoes	Extend shelf life
Dry or dehydrated enzyme preparations	Control insects and microorganisms
Pork carcasses or fresh non-cut processed cuts	Control Trichinella spiralis
Fresh fruit	Delay maturation
Dry or dehydrated enzyme preparations	Decontamination
Dry or dehydrated aromatic vegetable substances	Decontamination
Poultry	Control pathogens
Red meat	Control pathogens and prolong shelf life

Fresh shell eggs — Control Salmonella species

Food	Dose Permitted, kGy	Date of Rule
Spices, dry veg seasoning	30 (maximum)	7/15/63
Wheat, wheat powd	0.2-0.5	8/21/63
White potatoes	0.05-0.15	11/1/65
Dry or dehydrated enzyme preparations	10 (maximum)	6/10/85
Pork carc. or fresh non-cut processed cuts	0.3 (minimum)-1.0 (maximum)	7/22/85
Fresh fruit	1	4/18/86
Dry or dehydrated enzyme preparations	10	4/18/86
Dry or dehydrated aromatic vegetable substances	30	4/18/86
Poultry	3	5/2/90
Red meat	4.5 (fresh)-7 (frozen)	12/3/97
Fresh shell eggs	3.0	7/12/00

(*) USDA rules may have a different timeline.

Labeling

"All irradiated food sold in the United States must be clearly labeled with the international irradiation symbol, the Radura (Fig 1), and the words, "treated by irradiation, do not irradiate again" or "treated with radiation, do not irradiate again." The labeling law was amended in November 1997 and new labeling rules are currently in the public comment phase of rule making.

Figure 1

The Radura is the international symbol indicating a food product has been irradiated. All irradiated products sold in the United States since 1986 must carry the Radura. The Radura is usually green and resembles a plant in circle. The top half of the circle is dashed.

TAKING THE NEXT STEP

The Enviropig Has Arrived

"The "Enviropig" - a pig containing a novel trait expected to use plant phosphorus more efficiently - could reduce the negative environmental impact of high-density swine production. Researchers are taking a cautious approach to introducing these pigs onto the pork market, understanding the General public's wariness about genetically altered foods.

"Prof. Cecil Forsberg, graduate student Serguei Golovan, Department of Microbiology, and Prof. John Phillips, Department of Molecular Biology and Genetics, together with a team of researchers, have developed them. Of primary importance is the anticipated significant reduction of phosphorus found in their feces. Additional benefits may include improved utilization of minerals, protein and starch in the diet and the elimination of the need to supplement swine diets with phosphorous.

"By adding the blueprints of a bacterial enzyme into their genetic repertoire, the researchers have given a group of Yorkshire pigs the ability to extract phosphorus from the phytate molecule, a quality lacking in all other pigs with more being digested, less is wasted - a scenario that makes pigs' own "fertilizer" a little friendlier."

PIG CLONING PATENT FOR INFIGEN

"Infigen, Inc. (1825 Infinity Dr., DeForest, WI 53532; Tel: 608/846-0500; Website: www.infigen.com) has been awarded a major U.S. patent, entitled "Method of cloning porcine animals," covering the cloning of pigs using any porcine cell, including adult cells, and for the reprogramming of non-totipotent cells, or those otherwise unable to differentiate into other cells. U.S. Patent 6,258,998 also covers material relating to enhanced efficiencies for cloning pigs from all kinds of cells.

"Technology covered in this patent affords Infigen the ability to more easily produce cloned transgenic pigs as possible sources of replacement cells, tissues, and organs for xenotransplantation," says Michael Bishop, president and chief scientific officer of Infigen and one of the inventors named in the patent, along with Erik Forsberg and Jeffrey Betthauser, also Infigen employees.

"Separately, Infigen recently announced that it signed a 3-yr. collaboration with Immerge BioTherapeutics, a joint venture of Novartis Pharma AG (P.O. Box, CH-4002, Basel, Switzerland; Tel: +41 61 324 2476, Fax: 41 61 324-3300; Website: www.novartis.com) and BioTransplant, Inc. (Building 75, Third Ave.,

Charlestown Navy Yard, Charlestown, MA 02120; Tel: 617/241-5200, Fax: 617/241-8780) to use nuclear transfer (NT) technology to develop genetically modified miniature swine for the study of xenotransplantation (transplantation between species).

The Immerge BioTherapeutics/Infigen joint venture is cofunded by a Department of Commerce National Institute for Science and Technology (NIST). Infigen has produced the world's largest collection of cloned cows and pigs, more than 165 animals."

HOPE OR DOOM FOR ORGAN TRANSPLANT RECIPIENTS

"THE U.S. STAFF of PPL Therapeutics, Scotland, cloned five healthy female piglets, born on March 5, 2000, in Blacksburg, Virginia. This is the first time cloned pigs have been produced from adult pig cells.

"Their birth marks the first step in making genetically modified pigs whose organs and cells can be successfully transplanted into humans without being rejected by the human immune system. The process of xenotransplantation (the transfer of organs from one species to another) may one day solve the worldwide organ shortage problem."

WHAT THE MEDICAL AND THE RELIGIOUS COMMUNITY SAY

Health, a popular health magazine published in Mountain View, California, declared regarding trichinosis, "The disease is painful, as the worms enter the more active muscles, such as chest, heart, eyes, and tongue . . . 'Particularly disturbing, is the fact that the medical profession as a whole does not recognize this parasitic infection, but writes down a diagnosis of typhoid, intestinal flu, pleurisy, or may even operate for appendicitis. In all, some sixty diseases have been confused with trichinosis.' " (July, 1939.)

That trichinosis is caused by pork eating is abundantly evident from the following quotation. "Dr. Harry Most of New York University, asserted that in an examination of one hundred bodies in New York City, 'more than one out of five were infested with trichinae.' He added that in two hundred additional examinations of the diaphrams of orthodox and unorthodox Jews there was 'only one positive case.' "_Signs of the Times, March 11, 1941. Such findings from so large a number of examinations makes very apparent that few Jews have trichinosis, simply because they abstain from swine's flesh, according to the instruction of God penned in the Scriptures thousands of years ago.

"Should any feel disposed to claim that the Levitical law, regarding clean and unclean flesh foods, was given for the Jews only, we may then inquire is it not just as necessary that people of other nationalities escape the destructive trichina worm as it is that the Jews avoid becoming prey for the parasites? Surely the disease would cause the Jews no more suffering and pain than it would people of other nationalities."

"Pork or pig, all its parts and by-products, has been a chief food for most Americans, especially the Blacks since the days of their physical bondage. The pig was not made for human consumption. The pig is the chief cause of many of the ills and mental deficiencies occurring among them and any other people who eat it.

The pig is a mass of worms that are not nutritious at all. Each mouthful you eat is a mass of small worms, which the naked eye cannot detect. Worms thrive in the hog. When these worms are digested into your system, multiply to hundreds of new worms called larvae which travels the blood stream of your system and lodge in your muscles. These worms even enter your brain, lungs or your spinal fluid. They cause muscular aches, fever and many other symptoms of sickness. The worm has an amazing ability to go undetected in your system for many years. The scientific name for the ill-causing worm found in all pork is Trichinella spiralis, which causes trichinosis.

Regardless of what veterinarians, public health officials, the U.S. Agricultural Department or your doctor say, the best defense against the pig is NOT EATING IT! When you do eat it, you do not hurt God, the prophets, Jewish people, vegetarians, the Muslims or anyone else. You hurt yourself.

I am reminded of an experience when visiting my family. One of my relatives was talking to other relatives while circled in the living room. One stated boldly, "Well, I'd better get on home so I can soak those chittlins for the holidays. I soak mine in vinegar and salt." Of course, as she said this she looked quickly over at my wife and myself. My wife and I looked at each other and just about had to pinch one another to hold back the laughter and an attack in order to maintain the peace.

How often do we who understand the dangers of this rat tell our loved ones over and over to stay away from this animal. And how often do they try defending it without knowledge. My wife and I could have easily told her that even if she went home and soaked those (chittlins) intestines and "boo boo" track of that hog in high octane gasoline, then boiled them in nuclear acid, that would not free that hog meat of worms.

You are what you eat, so why not eat the best and be the best. Do not allow this rotten, diseased meat to be sold in your neighborhoods or brought into your homes.

While at my grandmother's house, she is very considerate of my family so much so, she actually has special dishes she gives us to use when we visit her. Her age and condition prevents her from eating the way she now understands she should; for her children - my aunts and uncles - still eat hog and still feed her the same.
How often have we heard the term, "cured" when it comes to that hog? The word "cured" is the past tense of the verb "cure." Here is a question you must ask yourself: If a meat has to be cured before we eat it, we should not even take the chance to eat it, because we have already told ourselves, thus admitting that it had to have been diseased at some point. Have we become so greedy for this particular meat that we are even willing to chance being poisoned from eating it? This sounds like the characteristics of a swine!

Not only in the Bible (book of the Christians and Jews), but as well in the Holy Qur-an (book of the Muslims), it is the Divine will of God that the pig should not be eaten and God has never changed this instruction. Just because the merchants of death, who sell drugs, whisky and other vice say it's all right, do you still indulge yourselves? Likewise, these same merchants have set up governmental bureaus to grade and approve the selling of pork.

"Strict Orthodox Jews follow the law that Allah gave to Moses on what food to eat and those strict Jews will not eat the prohibited foods that Allah made prohibited. So, their food is good for you, Allah teaches us in the Holy Qur-an. And, the strict Muslim food is good for the Jew.

"TOUCH NOT that which Allah has forbidden to be touched. There are many tricks that the [merchants are] playing on the total population in our foods and drinks so we have to be on our guard when we go to the market to purchase our food.

Pork destroys the beautiful appearance of its eaters. It takes away the shyness of those who eat this brazen flesh. Nature did not give the hog anything like shyness. You are what you eat. The eater takes on the characteristics of that which he eats.

"Take a look at their immoral dress and actions; their worship of filthy songs and dances that an uncivilized animal or savage human being of the jungle cannot even imitate....

"The Arabic meaning of hog, or swine, according to one Arab Muslim, is Khanzier. Khan, he says, means "I see." Zier means "foul." This is the meaning of the English word swine. Khanzier, or "I see the animal foul". And very foul is the best explanation that I have heard to cover the very nature and characteristics of this animal.

"The hog takes away the beautiful appearance of people and takes away their shyness. The people who eat the hog have no shyness because they eat the hog. Nature did not give the hog any shyness...The scientists have found that the hog carries 999 poisonous germs in it and they are not 100 percent poison, but nearly 1000 per cent poison. The swine takes away our life gradually and creates worms in our bodies.

"The worms eat away our digestive tracts and cause bad thinking, because once they get into the spinal cord, they make their way to the brain and there they begin to affect our way of thinking, until they have eaten your life away. They are parasitic worms, referred to as pork or trichina worms. They cannot be seen by the naked eye -- only under a microscope. They destroy three one-hundredths per cent of the beauty appearance of the eater, besides giving him fever, chills and headaches. Hayfever is also common among swine eaters."

Poultry Avian Influenza (Bird Flu)

Avian influenza is an infection caused by avian (bird) influenza (flu) viruses. These influenza viruses occur naturally among birds. Wild birds worldwide carry the viruses in their intestines, but usually do not get sick from them. However, avian influenza is very contagious among birds and can make some domesticated birds, including chickens, ducks, and turkeys, very sick and kill them.

Infected birds shed influenza virus in their saliva, nasal secretions, and feces. Susceptible birds become infected when they have contact with contaminated secretions or excretions or with surfaces that are contaminated with secretions or excretions from infected birds. Domesticated birds may become infected with avian influenza virus through direct contact with infected waterfowl or other infected poultry, or through contact with surfaces (such as dirt or cages) or materials (such as water or feed) that have been contaminated with the virus.

Infection with avian influenza viruses in domestic poultry causes two main forms of disease that are distinguished by low and high extremes of virulence. The “low pathogenic” form may go undetected and usually causes only mild symptoms (such as ruffled feathers and a drop in egg production). However, the highly pathogenic form spreads more rapidly through flocks of poultry. This form may cause disease that affects multiple internal organs and has a mortality rate that can reach 90-100% often within 48 hours.

Human infection with avian influenza viruses
There are many different subtypes of type A influenza viruses. These subtypes differ because of changes in certain proteins on the surface of the influenza A virus (hemagglutinin [HA] and neuraminidase [NA] proteins). There are 16 known HA subtypes and 9 known NA subtypes of influenza A viruses. Many different combinations of HA and NA proteins are possible. Each combination represents a different subtype. All known subtypes of influenza A viruses can be found in birds.

Usually, “avian influenza virus” refers to influenza A viruses found chiefly in birds, but infections with these viruses can occur in humans. The risk from avian influenza is generally low to most people, because the viruses do not usually infect humans. However, confirmed cases of human infection from several subtypes of avian influenza infection have been reported since 1997. Most cases of avian influenza infection in humans have resulted from contact with infected poultry (e.g., domesticated chicken, ducks, and turkeys) or surfaces contaminated with secretion/excretions from infected birds. The spread of avian influenza viruses from one ill person to another has been reported very rarely, and has been limited, inefficient and unsustained.

"Human influenza virus" usually refers to those subtypes that spread widely among humans. There are only three known A subtypes of influenza viruses (H1N1, H1N2, and H3N2) currently circulating among humans. It is likely that some genetic parts of current human influenza A viruses came from birds originally. Influenza A viruses are constantly changing, and they might adapt over time to infect and spread among humans.

During an outbreak of avian influenza among poultry, there is a possible risk to people who have contact with infected birds or surfaces that have been contaminated with secretions or excretions from infected birds.

Symptoms of avian influenza in humans have ranged from typical human influenza-like symptoms (e.g., fever, cough, sore throat, and muscle aches) to eye infections, pneumonia, severe respiratory diseases (such as acute respiratory distress), and other severe and life-threatening complications. The symptoms of avian influenza may depend on which virus caused the infection.

Studies done in laboratories suggest that some of the prescription medicines approved in the United States for human influenza viruses should work in treating avian influenza infection in humans. However, influenza viruses can become resistant to these drugs, so these medications may not always work.

Fish

The Messenger's dietary laws appear to be more lenient when it comes to fish, particularly because it comes from a different atmosphere; however, he does point out that even fish is not good for us due to their animal-like instincts in the water. But, we eat them and it is not a sin. He recommends that when eating them, restrict their weights from 1-1/2 to 5 pounds. Generally, larger fish are scavengers. The type of fish that are good or bad to eat are pointed out in his books. The instinct of the fish being a primary reason for not eating them has become an understatement with understanding the new dangers surrounding fish.

Mercury In Fish

Mercury is a mineral that exists naturally in the environment. In addition, thousands of tons are released into the air each year through pollution and waste. Bacteria and natural processes can transform mercury into the organic mercury compound methylmercury (MeHg), which is a poisonous substance.

Unfortunately, this toxin is in the fish we eat. Methylmercury can accumulate in streams and oceans. It also accumulates in the food chain, as each fish absorbs all the mercury of the smaller fish or organisms it has eaten. That is why the oldest and largest fish, such as shark or swordfish, have the highest levels.

Methylmercury levels are higher in people who regularly eat fish.

Who is at risk?

No one is immune to the potential dangers of high levels of mercury accumulated in their body tissues. The Centers for Disease Control and Prevention (CDC) reports that people most sensitive to mercury are pregnant and nursing women, children under the age of six (especially up to the age of three), people with impaired kidney function, and those with very sensitive immune responses to metals.

Methylmercury easily crosses the placenta and accumulates in the blood and tissues of the developing fetus. It can be passed to newborns through breast milk, and a baby's growing brain and nervous system are even more sensitive to this toxin than an adult's. Children remain particularly vulnerable for at least several years because, compared to adults, they eat more food relative to their body size.

According to a 2005 EPA study, women living in US coastal communities - and presumably eating more fish than inland residents do - had higher average blood levels of methylmercury. Women living on the Atlantic coast had the highest average levels, followed by women on the Pacific and then women on the Gulf coasts. Many had methylmercury levels that the EPA considers unsafe for adults.

Which fish are harmful? There is limited information about methylmercury in fish because there is no national or statewide system in place to monitor amounts. Most states, Native American tribes, and U.S. territories issue advisories that warn people when they are aware of methylmercury contamination. The advisories indicate what types, size, and amounts of fish are of concern. Pollution can result in high mercury levels in fish. Otherwise, methylmercury levels for many fish are relatively low, ranging from less than 0.01 part per million (ppm) to 0.5 ppm.

A few fish are so high in methylmercury that they should be totally avoided by pregnant or nursing women, young children, and other at-risk populations. In March 2004, the Food and Drug Administration (FDA) and the Environmental Protection Agency (EPA) issued a joint Consumer Advisory warning about methylmercury in fish. The advisory continues a previous warning against four particular species of fish and for the first time includes a specific warning about the consumption of tuna.

Is Farmed Raised Fish The Alternative?

The Food and Drug administration has given a clean bill of health to farm-raised fish in Washington state despite the discovery of toxic melamine in some of the feed used in the state's aquaculture industry.

The FDA report follows a scare over melamine-contaminated pet food that was blamed for causing the deaths of an unknown number of dogs and cats in the United States.

The earlier fears over contaminated feed are resurfacing concerns over aquaculture. Fish farms have struggled to improve their own image amid concerns about pollution and complaints about the flavor of the products they produce.

On harvest day at American Gold Seafood company in Puget Sound, thousands of fat Atlantic salmon are sucked up and sent flopping down plastic chutes, where they're funneled into a machine that delivers a pneumatic whack on the head, and a blade to the heart.

The manager, Rob Miller, is proud of this operation.
"These fish are stunned, bled and chilled in two hours, and (then) they're at the processing plant," explained Rob Miller, the plant's manager. "Within 12 hours we can have fresh filets ready to go."

Farmed salmon is cheap, and it's what most Americans eat. But it's also controversial: environmentalists don't like the pollution from the pens, and organic-minded consumers turn up their noses at what they perceive as an inferior flavor. So companies such as American

Gold have been trying to develop something they call "natural" farmed salmon.

The difference, Miller said, is the feed.

"In the natural feed there is no land animal protein. So all the protein sources come from either vegetable or fish," he said.

Miller said the theory is that since wild salmon eat fish, farmed salmon should eat feed made from fish. Even so, one of the feed brands used at American Gold may have been contaminated with melamine.

FDA tests show the fish themselves are free of the chemical, but critics of fish farming say the melamine scare should be taken as a warning.

"The important part of this is the feed process, right? Since we're industrializing the whole process of creating fish feed, there's a lot more opportunity for contaminants or problems to enter the system," said Andrea Kavanaugh, who directs the National Environmental Trust's "Pure Salmon" campaign.

In principle, Kavanaugh said she doesn't oppose fish farms. They're necessary to relieve pressure on the over-fished oceans, she said.

But she wants government regulations governing the operation of "organic" farmed salmon. Kavanaugh is also skeptical of the "natural" label being used to market the fish.

"I think that you can have a better, more sustainable, more environmentally friendly farmed salmon," she said, adding that the farmed salmon on the market is still far from "natural."

Miller readily admits "natural farmed salmon" is a vague concept.

"This is kind of a (fish) diet that we made up. Because there are no criteria for what should be in the 'natural' or 'organic' diets," he said.

As for the purists who refuse to eat farmed salmon, Miller likes to point out that many wild salmon start their lives in Washington state's hatcheries.

FRUITS & VEGETABLES (GENETICALLY ENGINEERED/ MODIFIED)

What are Genetically Modified (GM) Foods?

Although "biotechnology" and "genetic modification" commonly are used interchangeably, GM is a special set of technologies that alter the genetic makeup of such living organisms as animals, plants, or bacteria. Biotechnology, a more general term, refers to using living organisms or their components, such as enzymes, to make products that include wine, cheese, beer, and yogurt.

Combining genes from different organisms is known as recombinant DNA technology, and the resulting organism is said to be "genetically modified," "genetically engineered," or "transgenic." GM products (current or in the pipeline) include medicines and vaccines, foods and food ingredients, feeds, and fibers.

Locating genes for important traits—such as those conferring insect resistance or desired nutrients—is one of the most limiting steps in the process. However, genome sequencing and discovery programs for hundreds of different organisms are generating detailed maps along with data-analyzing technologies to understand and use them.

In 2003, about 167 million acres (67.7 million hectares) grown by 7 million farmers in 18 countries were planted with transgenic crops, the principal ones being herbicide- and insecticide-resistant soybeans, corn, cotton, and canola. Other crops grown commercially or field-tested are a sweet potato resistant to a virus that could decimate most of the African harvest, rice with increased iron and vitamins that may alleviate chronic malnutrition in Asian countries, and a variety of plants able to survive weather extremes.

On the horizon are bananas that produce human vaccines against infectious diseases such as hepatitis B; fish that mature more quickly; fruit and nut trees that yield years earlier, and plants that produce new plastics with unique properties.

In 2003, countries that grew 99% of the global transgenic crops were the United States (63%), Argentina (21%), Canada (6%), Brazil (4%), and China (4%), and South Africa (1%). Although growth is expected to plateau in industrialized countries, it is increasing in developing countries. The next decade will see exponential progress in GM product development as researchers gain increasing and unprecedented access to genomic resources that are applicable to organisms beyond the scope of individual projects.

Technologies for genetically modifying (GM) foods offer dramatic promise for meeting some areas of greatest challenge for the 21st century. Like all new technologies, they also poses some risks, both known and unknown. Controversies surrounding GM foods and crops commonly focus on human and environmental safety, labeling and consumer choice, intellectual property rights, ethics, food security, poverty reduction, and environmental conservation.

Controversies

Safety

Potential human health impact: allergens, transfer of antibiotic resistance markers, unknown effects Potential environmental impact: unintended transfer of transgenes through cross-pollination, unknown effects on other organisms (e.g., soil microbes), and loss of flora and fauna biodiversity

Access and Intellectual Property

Domination of world food production by a few companies
Increasing dependence on Industralized nations by developing countries

Biopiracy—foreign exploitation of natural resources

Ethics

Violation of natural organisms' intrinsic values
Tampering with nature by mixing genes among species
Objections to consuming animal genes in plants and vice versa
Stress for animal

Labeling

Not mandatory in some countries (e.g., United States)
Mixing GM crops with non-GM confounds labeling attempts
Society
New advances may be skewed to interests of rich countries

WHITE SUGAR

"...For carrying away any suspended protein matter that may remain, blood albumin from the slaughter house is used.

"Also purchased from the slaughter house is bone black or animal charcoal, which comes from low grade animals used as filter to 'purify' this mixture called sugar.

"It is then bleached with a strong bleaching agent referred to as blue water. This process holds true with first grade sugar but becomes much worse with low grade sugars.

"These inferior sugars are extracted from molasses by products by the action of strong chemicals such as calcium and barium hydroxide. This low grade sugar is what is used in gelatin, jams jellies, baking and bakery products.

"Commercial sugar is representative of the ultimate extreme in food degeneration. To just merely state that it is a starvation food is putting it very mildly. The term food is certainly a misnomer. Sugar is one of the most poisonous and injurious product in our Nation's diet with no exceptions and under every possible condition.

"These facts assume special importance when it is pointed out that more than sixty five percent of the animals slaughtered for the markets are swine. Therefore the slaughter house products being used in processing sugar are derivatives of pork."

"This certainly does not help the feelings of vegetarians who are deliberately trying hard to avoid the use of animal products and especially pork, I would venture to say the average vegetarian consumes at least one hog a year by eating sugar products without ever realizing it! Pig is in White Sugar and it's Products.

How To Eat To Live talks about sugar, but the Messenger says brown sugar is better. We want to make sure you understand which brown sugar he is referring to. He doesn't on one hand teaches us not to eat refined products and on the other suggest refined brown sugar the way it is produced today. KNOW THE DIFFERENCE. Raw brown sugar is what he means.

The Great Sugar Debate: Is it vegan?

Bone char, made from the bones of cows, is at times used to whiten sugar. Some sugar companies use it in filters to decolorize their sugar. Other types of filters involve granular carbon or an ion exchange system rather than bone char.

The following sugar companies DO NOT use bone-char filters:

Florida Crystals Refinery
P.O. Box 86
South Bay, FL 33493
407-996-9072
Labels: Florida Crystals

Refined Sugars Incorporated
One Federal St.
Yonkers, NY 10702
914-963-2400
Labels: Jack Frost, Country Cane, Flow-Sweet

Pillsbury
Makes powdered brown sugar
Supreme Sugar Company (subsidiary of Archer Daniels Midland)
P.O. Box 56009
New Orleans, LA 70156 504-831-0901
Labels: Supreme, Southern Bell, Rouse's Markets

The following sugar companies DO use bone-char filters:

Domino
1114 Ave. of the Americas
25th Fl.
New York, NY 10036
212-789-9700

Savannah Foods
P.O. Box 335
Savannah, GA 31402
912-234-1261

California & Hawaiian Sugar Company (with the exception of its Washed Raw Sugar)
830 Loring Ave.
Crockett, CA 94525-1104
510-787-2121

Supermarket brands of sugar (e.g., Giant, Townhouse, etc.) buy their sugar from several different refineries, so there is no way of knowing whether it is vegan at any given time.

Brown sugar is generally made by adding molasses to refined sugar, so sugar companies that use bone char in the production of their regular sugar will also use it in the production of their brown sugar. Confectioner's sugar (refined sugar mixed with cornstarch) made by such companies also involves the use of bone char. Fructose may, but does not typically involve a bone-char filter.

If you want to avoid all refined sugars, we recommend alternatives such as Sucanat and turbinado (RAW) sugar. Neither of these sweeteners are ever filtered with bone char. Additionally, beet sugar--though normally refined--never involves the use of bone char.

NATURAL BROWN (RAW) SUGAR

Natural brown sugar is a name for raw sugar which is a brown sugar produced from the first crystallisation of cane. Raw sugar is more commonly used, then further processed white sugar. As such "natural brown sugar" is free of additional dyes and chemicals. There is a higher level of inclusion of molasses than brown sugar giving it a higher mineral content. Some instances of natural brown sugars have particular names and characteristics and are sold as such: eg Demerara or Muscovado.

Why Is It Healthier?

Natural Brown Sugar is processed the natural way–completely free from any harmful chemicals such as phosphoric acid, formic acid, sulphur dioxide, preservatives, or any flocculants, surfactants, bleaching agents or viscosity modifiers.

Natural Brown Sugar has 11 calories/ 4 grams (1tsp). It is also nutritionally rich & retains all natural mineral & vitamin content present inherent in sugarcane juice.

Imbalance in minerals is one prime cause of disease. Reason for this is over- consumption of refined products like refined sugars, refined oils, & refined salt. It is therefore vital to consume less processed, more natural & nutritious products such as the healthy & wholesome Natural Brown Sugar.

Overall Comparisson

BROWN/ (DEMERARA)

Physical Appearance: Yellowish-brown sugar in the rich aroma of tropical sugarcane.

Production Process: Produced by a precise co-crystallization process to retain natural flavor & color components.

Chemical Additives: At no stage in the production process, are any chemical additives added. It is free from any harmful chemicals like phosphoric acid, formic acid, sulphur dioxide, preservatives /bleaching agents. This results in a health-friendly and chemical-free sugar.

Nutrition Content: Apart from a pure and natural sweetness, it contains 187 mg calcium, 56 mg phosphorous, 4.8mg iron, 757 mg potassium, and 97 mg sodium per cup of sugar-all from natural sources.

SUGAR: ORDINARY WHITE SUGAR

Physical Appearance: No flavor, taste, or color from natural sources.

Production Process: Ordinary sugar manufacture process employs several chemicals.

Chemical Additives: Processing involves a potpourri of chemicals; all finally showing their impact on our health in the long run. Sulphur carryover puts health at stake.

Nutrition Content: Does not contain natural minerals.

COOKING OIL

When it comes to cooking oil, the Messenger says that corn oil is good, but we must be mindful of current processes, which is one of the main reasons this book is being written. Corn oil of the 60's, for example, when How To Eat To Live was first published, is not the same as corn oil of today. Corn oil as well as canola and soy oil is being genetically altered for various purposes. One being that it has become an alternative energy source for fueling automobiles and secondly, it is being processed dangerously to feed world populations.

Canola Oil

The more research you do, the more you will see a relationship between the food you eat and fatal diseases. Canola oil is no exception. Reading our previous statements, you will be familiar with the meat industry practice of feeding rendered meat "by-products" to cattle and poultry, and the suspected relationship of Mad Cow Disease to CJD and Alzheimer's Disease. Now comes information that Canola Oil is the suspected causative agent for Scrapie, a viral disease transmitted to cattle who were fed rendered sheep infected with Scrapie. Both Scrapie and Mad Cow Disease destroy the brain's ability to function. They literally eat the brain away, causing blindness, loss of mind and erratic behavior.

Canola oil's real name is "LEAR" oil (Low Erucic Acid Rape). It is more commonly known as "rape oil," a semi-drying oil that is used as a lubricant, fuel, soap and synthetic rubber base, and as an illuminant to give color pages in magazines their slick look. In short it is an industrial oil that does not belong in the human body. It is typically referred to in light industry as a penetrating oil. Canola oil is a GM or genetically modified product. You have read about genetically modified foods previously.

In addition, a recent report from the EPA (1998) states that they have classified canola oil as a biopesticide, which ..."has low chronic toxicities". Further, they say that no studies have been done regarding toxic effects on Humans. The fact that they state that it is a pesticide and that there have been no studies, plus the fact it is a GM food, says to us it is something to stay away from! It is like so many other things "they" say are good for us like fluoride (to be addressed later), canola oil and fluoride both accumulate and build up in the Human systems.

Back in the 1980's, rape oil was widely used in animal feeds in England and throughout Europe. It was banned in 1991. Since then, Scrapie in sheep has totally disappeared.

While that's good for Europeans, it is bad for Americans, because the problem is now ours. Rape seed oil (Canola oil) is widely used in thousands of processed foods...with the blessings of our own government.

Canola oil was first developed in Canada. It's proponents claim that due to genetic engineering and irradiation (to be addressed later), it is no longer rape oil, but "canola" (Canadian oil). They also claim it is completely safe, pointing to it's unsaturated structure and digestibility. Although, this could not be verified, it is claimed the Canadian government paid the FDA the sum of $50 million dollars to have canola oil placed on the GRAS list (Generally Recognized As Safe). However it was done, a new industry was created.

The truth is however, that rape is the most toxic of all food oil plants. Not even insects will eat it. No wonder farmers like growing it. It turns out that rape is a member of the mustard family of plants, and is the source for the chemical agent, mustard gas, which causes blistering on skin and lungs when inhaled. Mustard Gas was banned after WWI for this very reason.

Studies of canola oil done on rats indicate many problems. Rats developed fatty degeneration of heart, kidney, adrenals and thyroid gland. When the canola oil was withdrawn from their diet, the deposits dissolved, but scar tissue remained on the organs. Why were no studies done on humans before the FDA placed it on the GRAS list?

Consumed in food, Canola oil depresses the immune system, causing it to "go to sleep." Canola oil is high in glycosides, which cause health problems by blocking (inhibiting) enzyme function. Its effects are accumulative, taking years to show up. One possible effect of long-term use is the destruction of the protective coating surrounding nerves called the myelin sheath. When this protective sheath is gone, our nerves short-circuit causing erratic, uncontrollable movements.
To test the industrial penetrating strength of canola oil, soak a towel in both canola oil and regular vegetable oil. Pre-treat and wash the towel in your clothes washer and compare the area the two oils occupied...you will notice an oil stain remains on the area soaked in canola oil. It is so durable, it could take several washings to completely remove. Now if this is how canola oil penetrates the fabric of a towel, what damage can it do in your body?

Because canola oil is so cheap, it is now widely used in the food industry. If you are curious, just read a few food labels the next time you are in the grocery store. A good example can be found with commercially prepared peanut butter. In order to give peanut butter it's spreadability, peanut butter companies remove ALL of the natural peanut oil and replace it with canola oil. Natural peanut butter should only have peanuts and salt listed in the ingredients.

Food consumers have headaches enough, without worrying about a toxic plant oil being added to their food. The problem is you will find canola oil in bread, margarines, and all manner of processed foods including potato chips. But the consumer is king. Be informed and make it a practice to read the package ingredients label as to what is in the food. Avoid using canola as a cooking oil and salad oil. It is not a healthy oil. It'll work great for lubricating mechanical items.

What We Do:

Pure Olive oil is best, as taught by Messenger Elijah Muhammad.

Bear in mind that oils containing Omega 6, which is not a good option for the heart or the mylin sheaths, should be avoided as well. We automatically reject any foods, packaged or otherwise, which have in the label "...may contain vegetable oil, cottonseed, canola oil.." And if the label just says vegetable oil, we reject it outright since it does not specify which oil.

HOW TO RECOGNIZE ORGANIC VERSUS GENETICALLY MODIFIED FRUITS & VEGETABLES

While unpacking groceries, you pull out the bag of apples and decide to eat one then and there. You take it over to the sink, wash it off and -- with some effort -- peel off the little sticker. Pausing to look more closely at the sticker you wonder, "What do those numbers mean?"

As much as we may dislike them, the stickers or labels attached to fruit do more than speed up the scanning process at the checkout stand. The PLU code, or price lookup number printed on the sticker, tells you how the fruit was grown.

By reading the PLU code, you can tell if the fruit was genetically modified, organically grown or produced with chemical fertilizers, fungicides, or herbicides.

Labeling Standards: North America

General designation is as follows:

Organic produce has a five-digit number beginning with a 9. Organic bananas, for example, would be given the designation of 94011.

Conventional produce has a four-digit number beginning with a 3 or 4. Therefore, the number on conventionally grown bananas would be 4011. For conventionally grown fruit, (grown with chemicals inputs), the PLU code on the sticker consists of four numbers.

Genetically engineered produce also has a five-digit number on the label and begins with an 8. Again, the number on genetically altered bananas would be 84011.

The numeric system was developed by the Produce Electronic Identification Board, an affiliate of the Produce Marketing Association, a Newark, Delaware-based trade group for the produce industry. As of October 2001, the board had assigned more than 1,200 PLUs for individual produce items.

Incidentally, the adhesive used to attach the stickers is considered food-grade, but the stickers themselves aren't edible.

Do you REALLY know what's in your dinner?

Today, 7 out of every 10 items on grocery stores shelves contain ingredients that have been genetically modified. In other words, scientists are using new technology to transfer the genes of one species to another, and these altered foods are in the market stream. And yet many scientists have concerns about the safety -- to people, wildlife and the environment -- of this process. That's why consumers in Asia and

Europe are demanding that their food be free of genetically modified ingredients.

How To Eat To Live, are revolutionary books written before their time. Elijah Muhammad never said that Allah is the only knower, just THE BEST KNOWER.

Most Produce Look-Up numbers (PLU) consist of four digits. They are mainly used in supermarkets to identify fruits and vegetables at the check-out.

Some four-digit PLUs are prefixed with an 8 (8xxxx) which denotes genetically modified produce and a 9 (9xxxx) which denotes organically grown produce. Both numbers are prefixes to the standard four digit PLU numbers.

An excellent reference source is that of the International Federation for Produce Coding at http://plu.plucodes.com/plucoding5/. You will need to fill in four question boxes in order to gain entry to the data tables. The questions are not personal or invasive of privacy.

You will find extensive tables of PLU numbers. Another source is at http://www.innvista.com/HEALTH/foods/plucodes_123.htm

The following listing comprises all those numbers and their associated fruits for which data was available in the alphabetical lists of labels.

3010 SUNDOWNER AUSTRALIAN ORIGINAL AND BEST []
3027 Jaffa SHAMOUTI []
3029 OUTSPAN Satsuma [orange]
3029 Satsuma [satsuma]
3030 Forbel Nova [clementine]
3030 LAFAL CYPRIA MANDARIN
3030 MANDARIN
3031 CYPRIA MANDORA []
3031 Jaffa MANDOR []
3031 OUTSPAN Tambor [orange]
3032 Ellendale [orange]
3107 Dole Navel [orange]
3107 Navel
3107 OUTSPAN Navel []
3108 OUTSPAN Valencia []
3111 Caliman PAPAYA BRAZIL
3153 DELTA SEEDLESS []
3155 Midknight
4011 Bonita Ecuador [banana]
4011 Del Monte Quality R [banana]
4011 PRATT'S COSTA RICA [banana]
4011 SCB CÔTE D'IVOIRE Premium
4012 Large Navel [orange]

HOW TO RECOGNIZE ORGANIC VERSUS GENETICALLY MODIFIED FRUITS & VEGETABLES

4012 OUTSPAN Navelate []
4015 Cape Late Top Red [apple]
4015 RED DELICIOUS [apple]
4015 TOP RED SOUTH AFRICA [apple]
4015 WASHINGTON RED DELICIOUS [apple]
4017 GRANNY SMITH [apple]
4021 Cape GOLDEN [apple]
4021 COX RICH AND AROMATIC [apple]
4021 COX [apple]
4021 Dole Navel [navel orange]

4021 Golden Delicious FRANCE [apple]
4021 GOLDEN DELICIOUS SWEET JUICY [apple]
4021 Goldens South Africa [apple]
4021 HOCHLAND GOLDENS
4024 Green Williams [pear]
4030 Clée [kiwifruit]
4030 Copefrut KIWIFRUIT
4030 Kiwifruit [kiwifruit]
4030 Zespri NEW ZEALAND [kiwifruit]
4030 [kiwifruit]
4032 [melon]
4042 Chiquita [banana]
4051 El Tropico [mango]
4051 Master's Touch [mango??]
4051 PANGO MANGO USA [mango]
4053 ASDA Lemons PLU4053
4059 Copefrut KIWIFRUIT
4101 Braeburn France [apple]
4101 Braeburn Fresh and Crunchy [apple]
4101 BRAEBURN [apple]
4101 WASHINGTON BRAEBURN 4101 [apple]

4103 BRAEBURN [apple]
4105 enza COX ORANGE [apple]
4128 Pink Lady Australian[apple]
4128 STEMILT Pink Lady RESPONSIBLE CHOICE [apple]
4131 SUN MOON FUJI [apple]
4133 FISCHER GALA PRODUCE OF BRAZIL [apple]
4133 GALA SOUTH AFRICA [apple]
4139 COPEFRUT GRANNY SMITH [apple]
4139 enza Granny Smith [apple]
4139 GRANNY SMITH #4139 FRESH & TANGY [apple]
4167 RED DELICIOUS [apple]
4173 Copefrut ROYAL GALA [apple]
4173 enza ROYAL GALA NEW ZEALAND [apple]
4173 ROYAL GALA [apple]
4174 Cape ROYAL GALA [apple]
4174 enza ROYAL GALA NEW ZEALAND [apple]
4174 Royal Gala FRANCE [apple]
4174 Royal Gala SOLER
4186 SCB CÔTE D'IVOIRE Small bananas
4235 Banacol [banana]
4235 Del Monte Quality c [plantain]
4288 Best STAR RUBY Red Grapefruit
4288 Jaffa RED GRAPEFRUIT SUNRISE
4288 OUTSPAN STAR RUBY Red Grapefruit
4288 OUTSPAN Tambor [orange]
4291 Jaffa o [grapefruit]
4294 YELLOW GRAPEFRUIT
4317 Dole GOLDEN MELON
4382 Tomango [orange]
4383 Minneolas []
4408 Asian Pear
4408 NASHI PEAR [pear]

4413 McDonald Beurre Bosc [pear]
4414 Comice [pear]
4416 D'ANJOU SF Co []
4418 cape FORELLE [pear]
4418 Forelle [pear]
4421 Cape PACKHAM'S [pear]
4421 Packhams [pears]
4428 SHARONI [sharon fruit]
4428 [persimmon = sharon fruit]
4450 Clementine [clementine]
4450 OUTSPAN Clementine
4553 enza TAYLORS GOLD NEW ZEALAND [pear]

94129 WASHINGTON FUJI S Certified Organic [apple]

SHEA BUTTER

Shea nut butter maybe slightly greenish or ivory in color. It is a natural fat extracted from fruit of the Shea tree by crushing and boiling. Shea butter is widely used in cosmetics as a moisturizer and an emollient. Shea butter is also edible. It is used as a cooking oil in West Africa.

Types

There are two types of shea butter Certified Organic Unrefined and the Refined Version. The first is extracted using traditional extraction methods without the use of hexane, chemical pesticides, or preservatives. Because of this, many of the healing factors are still present in this form of shea butter. Refined Shea butter has been bleached, and refined with various chemicals such as hexane, fillers, and preservatives lacks many of the vital nutrients, phytochemicals and superb and powerful healing fraction of 100 % Pure Unrefined Certified Organic Shea Butter.

While a clean extracted butter is best for its overall healing ability, some may prefer a cosmetic grade butter that has been highly refined of impurities and aroma, although most of the natural properties and abilities of shea butter are stripped away when refined and it is much less effective and versatile than the unrefined butter.

Most commercialy available shea butter on the market is refined using fullers clay and a vacuum extraction method to eliminate shea butter's unpleasing aroma. However, the aroma of unrefined shea butter disappears within minutes as the butter absorbs into the skin. Shea butter is known commercially as Butyrospermum Parkii.

Unrefined shea butter contains an abundance of healing ingredients, including vitamins, minerals, proteins and a unique fatty acid profile, and is a superior active moisturizer. Unlike petroleum based moisturizers, shea butter actually restores the skin's natural elasticity. Shea butter actually enables your skin to absorb moisture from the air, and as a result, it becomes softer and stays moisturized for longer. In addition, shea butter has natural sunscreen properties and anti-inflammatory agents. Because of its amazing properties, shea butter is an excellent ingredient for soaps, lotions and creams. Perhaps it is most effective when applied to the skin in its pure state. Regular users of pure, unrefined shea butter notice softer, smoother,. healthier skin. Shea butter has also been shown to help with skin conditions and ailments such as extreme dryness, eczema, dermatitis, skin allergies, fungal infections, blemishes, wrinkles, stretch marks, scars, scrapes, and more.

Only pure, unrefined shea butter has the true healing and moisturizing properties of shea butter. Most shea butter available to the general public outside West Africa is white and odorless, in other words it has been "refined" to remove the natural scent and color of natural shea butter. In the process, the majority of the effective agents are also removed. In addition, refined shea butter has usually been extracted from the shea kernels with hexane or other petroleum solvents. The extracted oil is boiled to drive off the toxic solvents, and then refined, bleached, and deodorized, which involves heating it to over 400¡F and the use of harsh chemicals, such as sodium hydroxide. Shea butter extracted in this manner still contains some undesirable solvent residues, and its healing values are significantly reduced. Antioxidants or preservatives such as BHA (butylated hydroxyanisole) or BHT (butylated hydroxytoluene) may be added as well. The end result is an odorless, white butter that may be aesthetically appealing, but lacks the true moisturizing, healing, and no odor.nutritive properties of true traditional shea butter. In addition, refined shea butter is often hard and grainy, not smooth and creamy like pure, unrefined shea butter. All that can be said for refined shea butter is that it has an extended shelf life, a white, uniform color, and

EQUIPMENT

Cookware & Bakeware

There are many types of cookware and bakeware on the market--some tried and true, others brand new. Here's a rundown of what's currently available in my order of preference, with with regard to their health and environmental pros and cons.

Soapstone

Soapstone cookware is heavy, thick, and somewhat expensive, but it is an excellent conductor of heat. I am amazed at how quickly it will boil water, even at medium low heat. Soapstone cookware is energy-saving and will last several lifetimes, so it can be handed down from generation to generation. My soapstone pot is my favorite all-purpose cooking vessel.

Soapstone is a quarried stone like granite and marble. Its primary components are magnesite, dolomite, chlorite, and talc. The talc gives it the smooth feeling of rubbing a piece of dry soap--thus the name "soapstone."

Because it can be easily cut to shape without special stone cutting tools, soapstone has been used for thousands of years throughout the world for tools, karafes, vases, goblets, sinks, and other useful household objects.

Soapstone has many desirable qualities for cookware. It:

- is long lasting
- has no odor nor taste
- holds heat for long periods
- is virtually non-stick
- is beautiful enough to be used for serving
- will keep food hot during serving
- is completely non-porous, so it won't stain or hold food odors
- is bacteria resistant.

Glass (Best Choice)

The most popular glass cookware and bakeware is Pyrex (is there any other?), which has been in use for almost a century. Made by Corning Glass Works, the "low-expansion" glass was originally developed in response to a request from the railroads to produce lantern glass that would not break when the hot glass was struck by rain or snow. The super-tough "fire glass" was not only resistant to temperature fluctuations, but also chemical corrosion and breakage as well.

In 1913, the wife of one of Corning's scientists used a new casserole dish only twice before it fractured in the oven. Having heard about the glass her husband worked with, she asked him to bring home a fire-glass container she could use for baking. She baked a sponge cake and found the cooking time was shorter, the cake did not stick to the glass, the baking was unusually uniform, the flavor of the cake did not remain in the dish after washing, and she could watch the cake bake and know it was done by looking at the underside. These features have made Pyrex glass a favorite among home cooks.

According to their website, silica (a compound found in quartz and sand) is the main ingredient. "Eight ingredients are added and some broken glass" and all are cooked in a huge furnace at 3,000 degrees Fahrenheit. So while it doesn't contain recycled glass bottles, broken glass within the factory is recycled back into the pot. Pyrex is durable (so it can be reused for years without breaking or chipping) and it saves energy (Pyrex glass absorbs, rather than reflecting oven heat waves, thereby reducing cooking time over earthenware, porcelain or enameled dishes).
Pyrex is completely inert and does not leach anything into the food being cooked; you can bake and serve in the same dish, and then put it in the refrigerator and freezer.

Pyrex is affordable, comes in many sizes and shapes, and is sold everywhere.
Corning also makes tempered-glass Visions pots (made from a proprietary blend of glass and ceramic). Corning Visions is sold on the Internet and is available used on eBay and can often be found in thrift stores and flea markets.

Copper

Copper heats quickly and has very even heat distribution, so it is the choice of chefs everywhere. Copper will leach into food if you

cook in it directly, so most copper pots are lined (sugar pots for candymaking are not).
Today, most copper pots are lined with stainless steel, a manmade concoction of various metals that do not occur together in nature, and leach into food and water once the surface is scratched (see Stainless Steel below). Traditionally, copper pots were lined with tin, which is a natural element of the earth and considered to be the most inert of metals. Copper itself is also a naturally-occuring metal. Tin-lined copper pots are still available today, such as those made by Ruffoni.

Silicone

Silicone is now being used to make a whole variety of useful non-stick cooking items. They are bright and colorful and easy to store. While there are no stovetop pots and pans, there are hundreds of useful kitchen items, including baking pans, baking sheets, spatulas, molds, ice cube trays in fun shapes (that also can double for baking little cakes), rolling pins, and more.

Silicone is a synthetic polymer made from silica and other ingredients. Silica is common sand, made up of silicon, the second most abundant element in the earth's crust (about 28%). Silicon is not found in its elemental form but occurs mainly as oxides and silicates, like sand.

Silicones are made chemically by creating a "backbone" of silicon and oxygen molecules, a combination that does not occur in nature.

Then various other synthetic molecules are added branching off of the main silicon-oxygen line to create hundreds of different silicones that range from liquids to rubbery solids.
Trying to find some information on the health effects of silicone rubber is hard because it may not be listed in some of the toxic chemical databases consumers use.

Cooking with the cookware is very easy. Nothing sticks to them and they are very easy to clean. Silicone baking mats (which can be reused more than 2000 times) can save yards and yards of parchment paper!

Silicone has many desirable benefits:

- inherently nonstick without an added finish
- does not retain odors or flavors
- stain resistant
- dishwasher safe

can go from temperature extremes of -58 degrees F up to 428 degrees F, from freezer to oven [note home ovens can go up to 500 degrees F, so keep the 428 degree F limit in mind]

- promotes even heat distribution
- quick cooling
- some items can be folded for easy storage

Cast iron

Cast iron has been the mainstay cookware for generations. It's durable, inexpensive, and simple in materials, has even heating and good heat retention. But there is some controversy over the safety of the iron that may be released into the food. Some say it's a nutrient, or at least that it's harmless, others say the form of iron that is released is toxic. Regardless, it has been used for decades with no proven side effects.

Stainless steel

Stainless steel is generally considered the best choice for cooking because it is sanitary, nonporous, and the metals are highly stable. Environmentally, however, the mining and manufacture of steel is a highly technological, energy-intensive and polluting process. **Stainless steel also leaches nickel and chromium into food, which may be harmful to health**.

If you choose stainless steel for its advantages, then buy an energy-efficient brand to balance out some of the environmental disadvantages. This type of stainless steel cookware generally has double-walled sides and insulated lids allow you to slow-cook at lower temperatures and save a substantial amount of energy. In addition, because the pots retain heat, foods will continue to cook even after the pot is removed from the burner.

You can minimize the leaching of metals by only using wooden utensils in stainless steel pots and pans. **Metal utensils scratch the surface and release more metals**.

Aluminum

Aluminum salts from cookware can leach from the pot into the food being cooked, particularly if it is acidic, causing a number of unpleasant symptoms. The sale of aluminum-lined cookware is prohibited in Germany, France, Belgium, Great Britain, Switzerland, Hungary, and Brazil, but still permitted in America.

Most aluminum cookware manufactured today is anodized. When a cookware label says it is made from anodized aluminum, it means that the aluminum was dipped into a hot acid bath that seals the aluminum by changing its molecular structure.
If you buy used cookware at flea markets or thrift shops, however, check the label carefully and watch out for non-anodized aluminum. Non-anodized aluminum pots are usually heavy and look like they are pressed from a single piece of thick metal. The inside is the same color as the outside. Don't buy these.

There are some brands of cookware that use aluminum for the base of the pan because it distributes heat evenly and is relatively inexpensive, and then line the pan with stainless steel or some other finish. Cookware containing aluminum is safe to use only when the aluminum does not come in contact with the food, but those lined with stainless steel would have the same leaching problem as any stainless steel cookware.

Non-stick and porcelain enamel finishes

The problem with most non-stick finishes (such as Teflon) is that they are made from plastics that are simply a coating on an aluminum pan, so they chip and scratch easily and can contaminate your food. There is a new type, however, which locks the non-stick plastic finish into a crater-like material made from indestructable ceramic and titanium. Embedding the finish in the ceramic-titanium craters prevents it from being scraped off into the food, but fumes may still be released, especially as a result of long periods of excessive heat.

A recent investigation by the Environmental Working Group found that an independent science panel advised the EPA that Teflon is a "likely human carcinogen." The report says there is evidence that the manufacturer Dupont knew that Teflon was toxic, that it entered the bloodstream of people who used it, and that it is very persistent in the environment. Dupont is also undergoing a federal criminal investigation for allegedly suppressing studies regarding birth defects and other health hazards from Teflon.

Porcelain enamel finishes are completely inert and safe to use, but they also chip easily. **Slow cookers and crock pots use this coating.**

If you want a no-stick pan, get soapstone cookware, which is naturally non-stick, or get a cast iron pan and "season" it. Before using the cast iron pan, brush the bottom with cooking oil and place it in an oven at 400 degrees for about 20 to 40 minutes – depending on oven. Electric, for example is quicker. Wipe out the excess oil, leaving a thin film of oil on the pan. This process will leave a baked on oil coating in the pan.

METHODS: HEALTHY COOKING TIPS

- Always have a live Aloe Vera plant in the kitchen for accidental burns.
- Salt is a great purifier. Always wash raw fruits and vegetables in salted water before eating.
- To make garlic oil, chop 1 bulb of garlic and place inside of a glass jar, add 1 cup of extra virgin olive oil close with a lid to keep fresh and aromatic. Leave on counter to flavor other food. For the best garlic bread ever, brush on a little of this oil on toast.
- Always in a hurry, wash salad vegetables in salted water, place individual servings in quart size freezer bags and place in the refrigerator. When ready for a quick salad, just place a serving in a bowl and add dressing.
- When freezing fresh vegetables, make sure their not over ripe because the enzymes in them will continue the ripening process.
- To ripen fruit, place inside a plastic bag.
- Store olive oil in dark glass containers away from heat.
- Coffee, herbs and spices should be stored in the refrigerator. They will still be fresh past expiration date.
- When cleaning cookware, use borax, baking soda or sand from you back yard, pots and pans will shine like new.

- Peppermint tea is excellent for acid indigestion.
- Keep box of baking soda new stove to extinguish possible fires.

Always keep a things to do or shopping list attached to the refrigerator and write down items as soon as they run out to avoid trying to remember later.

GUIDE TO HEALTHY HOME PRODUCTS

Borax (booster, multipurpose cleaner & more)

What Is Borax?

Borax (also known as sodium borate decahydrate; sodium pyroborate; birax; sodium tetraborate decahydrate; sodium biborate) is a natural mineral compound ($Na2B4O7 \cdot 10H2O$). It was discovered over 4000 years ago. Borax is usually found deep within the ground, although it has been mined near the surface in Death Valley, California since the 1800s. Although it has numerous industrial uses, in the home borax is used as a natural laundry booster, multipurpose cleaner, fungicide, preservative, insecticide, herbicide, disinfectant, dessicant, and ingredient in making 'slime'. Borax crystals are odorless, whitish (can have various color impurities), and alkaline. Borax is not flammable and is not reactive. It can be mixed with most other cleaning agents, including chlorine bleach.

How Does Borax Clean?

Borax has many chemical properties that contribute to its cleaning power. Borax and other borates clean and bleach by converting some water molecules to hydrogen peroxide ($H2O2$). This reaction is more favorable in hotter water. The pH of borax is about 9.5, so it produces a basic solution in water, thereby increasing the effectiveness of bleach and other cleaners. In other chemical reactions, borax acts as a buffer, maintaining a stable pH needed to maintain cleansing chemical reactions. The boron, salt, and/or oxygen of boron inhibit the metabolic processes of many organisms. This characteristic allows borax to disinfect and kill unwanted pests. Borates bonds with other particles to keep ingredients dispersed evenly in a mixture, which maximizes the surface area of active particles to enhance cleaning power.

Risks Associated with Borax

Borax is natural, but that does not mean it is automatically safer for you or for 'the environment' than man-made chemicals. Although plants need boron, too much of it will kill them, so borax can be used as an herbicide. Borax may also be used to kill roaches, ants, and fleas. In fact, it is also toxic to people. Signs of chronic toxic exposure include red and peeling skin, seizures, and kidney failure. The estimated lethal dose (ingested) for adults is 15-20 grams; less than 5 grams can kill a child or pet. For this reason, borax should not be used around food. More commonly, borax is associated with skin, eye, or respiratory irritation. It is also important to point out that exposure to borax may impair fertility or cause damage to an unborn child.

Now, none of these risks mean that you shouldn't use borax. If you do a bit of research, you will find risks associated with all cleaning products, natural or man-made. However, you do need to be aware of product risks so that you can use those products properly. Don't use borax around food, keep it out of reach of children and pets, and make sure you rinse borax out of clothes and off of surfaces before use.

What You Need To Know About Borax

Borax is best known as a laundry booster; it helps soften hard water to leave your clothes cleaner and brighter. Your mother or grandmother probably kept a box of Borax in their laundry room. Well, it's time to rediscover the many safe, non-toxic household uses of Borax. From disinfecting and deodorizing to preserving cut flowers, Borax is a product you will want to keep on hand at all times.
How Safe is Borax
Borax has no toxic fumes and is safe for the environment.
Buy Borax Here20 Mule Team Borax,

What Does Borax Do?

- cleans
- deodorizes
- disinfects
- softens water
- repels cockroaches and other bugs

Bath Soap (See recommended sites in rear)

IT'S ALL IN YOUR HEAD

Metal In Your Mouth (Mercury)

Dental Amalgams the "silver" fillings in your teeth: Is It Safe?

Dental amalgam, the material in "silver" tooth fillings, contains approximately 50 per cent of the highly toxic heavy metal mercury. But is it safe to put so much Mercury, the most toxic non-radioactive metal known to man, into the mouth of a person?

The "silver" fillings in your teeth - Dental Amalgams - are still widely used by the dental profession in most parts of the world. The "Amalgam" consists of a mix of metals - Generally 50% Mercury, 35% Silver, 15% Tin and other metals. But is it safe to put so much Mercury, the most toxic non-radioactive metal known to man, into the mouth of a person?

There is now a growing mountain of evidence that it is NOT safe to do so. Some countries, like Sweden, Canada and Germany, have either banned or imposed serious limitations on Amalgam usage. There is now compelling evidence from reputable scientific bodies such as the World Health Organization that, despite claims from pro-amalgam bodies such as the

American and British Dental Associations (ADA/BDA), mercury is NOT "locked" safely in the metal bonds in the teeth, but can leak slowly into the body, often causing severe illnesses. These are reckoned to possibly include ME/CFS, Multiple Sclerosis, Alzheimers, and a whole range of "auto-immune" illnesses. In fact, just by damaging the immune system, Amalgam could be contributing to an even broader range of illnesses. Even dental floss has mercury and thallium on it.

IS DENTAL AMALGAM SAFE?

Mercury's extreme cytotoxicity and neurotoxicity is a major factor in the neurological conditions, along with its inhibition of basic enzymatic cellular processes and effects on essential minerals and nutrients in cells. Mercury is also documented to cause imbalances in neurotransmitters related to mood disorders. A direct mechanism involving mercury's inhibition of cellular enzymatic processes by binding with the hydroxyl radical(SH) in amino acids appears to be a major part of the connection to allergic/immune reactive conditions such as autism, schizophrenia, lupus, eczema and psoriasis, scleroderma, and allergies. Immune reactivity to mercury has been documented by immune reactivity tests to be a major factor in many of the autoimmune conditions.

We have discussed the two most common sources of toxic mercury: seafood and dental amalgams. But there's a third source of mercury that you should know about, particularly if you are the parent or grandparent of a young child or are expecting to have a child: vaccines.

Until recently, a form of mercury called thimerosal was used as a preservative in many of the vaccines given to infants and young children, including vaccines for hepatitis B, influenza, diphtheria, tetanus, pertussis, and Haemophilus influenzae type b (Hib). Congressman Dan Burton (R-Indiana), who spoke before the House Committee on Government Reform's hearing on mercury and medicine last year, knows just what this poison can do to the delicate brain and nervous system of a young child: his once-healthy grandson, who was given vaccines for nine different diseases in one day, now suffers from autism. In Burton's estimation, his grandson may have received, in the space of a few hours, 41 times the amount of mercury at which harm can be caused. Unfortunately, his grandson's experience is not unique.

Human destiny is on a collision course with mercury. Tomorrow we will all wake up to a world with about twenty tons more mercury in the environment, another ton will be put into people's mouths by dentists, and tens of thousands of little children will receive vaccinations laced with toxic mercury molecules, in the form of ethyl-mercury, supercharged with aluminum. In a world rapidly approaching some saturation point with mercury these twenty tons are significant. The longer medical and governmental authorities deny the full mercury story the higher the tide will rise as concentrations increase on land, sea and air. Mercury is a reality that has to be taken into account by doctors and everyone else.

Though mercury is accompanied by tens of thousands of other chemicals in the environment none are as toxic nor as prevalent. We are destroying our children and our future with an invisible enemy as surely as if we have fought and lost a nuclear war.

Mercury Destroys Brain Cells

As mentioned in the newsletter, mercury is a neurotoxin that is especially damaging to the developing brain and nervous system. A growing number of researchers believe that the soaring rates of neurological and developmental disorders in our children can be linked to a corresponding increase in the number of government-mandated vaccines.

The number of compulsory vaccines has increased from 10 to 36 in the past quarter-century, and over that time period, there has been a simultaneous increase in the number of children suffering from disabilities that prevent them from reaching their full potential. The incidence of learning disabilities and attention deficit disorder has doubled in the past 25 years, while autism has increased by an incredible 200 to 500 percent in every state in the U.S. in just the last decade.

Unnatural Chemicals associated with dental products.

- Mercury & Thallium Dental floss
- Cobalt Mouth wash
- Nickel Metal tooth filings & Retainers
- Titanium Metal dental ware
- Tin & Strontium Toothpaste
- Ytterbium, Erbium & +Terbium Plastic tooth fillings
- Benzalkonium & Zirconium Toothpaste & mouthwash
- Solvents Peroxide (store bought) Hydrogen Peroxide (Food-grade recommended)

HYDROGEN PEROXIDE – CURSE OR CURE?

By Dr. David G. Williams;

When it comes to hydrogen peroxide therapy, there seems to be only two points of view. Supporters consider it one of the greatest healing miracles of all time. Those opposed feel its ingestion is exceptionally dangerous, and only the foolhardy could think of engaging in such behavior. Before either condemning or endorsing hydrogen peroxide, let's take a real close look at what we're dealing with.

If any substance is interesting, it's hydrogen peroxide. Hydrogen peroxide should really be called hydrogen dioxide. Its chemical formula is H2O2. It contains one more atom of oxygen than does water (H20)

By now everyone's aware of the ozone layer that surrounds the earth. Ozone consists of three atoms of oxygen (03). This protective layer of ozone is created when ultraviolet light from the sun splits an atmospheric oxygen molecule (02) into two single, unstable oxygen atoms.

These single molecules combine with others to form ozone (03). Ozone isn't very stable. In fact, it will quickly give up that extra atom of oxygen to falling rainwater to form hydrogen peroxide

(FG-H2O2). (Bear with me: all this chemistry mumbo jumbo I'm going through actually will help you understand the importance of hydrogen peroxide.)

It is this hydrogen peroxide in rainwater that makes it so much more effective than tap water when given to plants. With the increased levels of atmospheric pollution, however, greater amounts of FG-H2O2 react with air-borne toxins and never reach the ground.

To compensate for this, many farmers have been increasing crop yields by spraying them with diluted hydrogen peroxide (5 to 16 ounces of 35% mixed with 20 gallons of water per acre).

You can achieve the same beneficial effect with your house plants by adding 1 ounce of 3% hydrogen peroxide (or 16 drops of 35% solution) to every quart of water you give your plants. (It can also be made into an excellent safe insecticide. Simply spray your plants with 8 ounces of 3% peroxide mixed with 8 ounces of white sugar and one gallon of water.)

Hydrogen peroxide is odorless and colorless, but not tasteless. When stored under the proper conditions, it is a very stable compound. When kept in the absence of light and contaminants, it dismutates (breaks down) very slowly at the rate of about 10% a year.

(This can be slowed even further by storing the liquid in the freezer.) It boils at 152 degrees C and freezes at minus 2 degrees C.
When exposed to other compounds hydrogen peroxide dismutates readily. The extra oxygen atom is released leaving H20 (water). In nature oxygen (02) consists of two atoms--a very stable combination.
A single atom of oxygen, however, is very reactive and is referred to as a free radical. Over the past several years, we've continually read that these free radicals are responsible for all types of ailments and even premature aging. What many writers seem to forget, however, is that our bodies create and use free radicals to destroy harmful bacteria, viruses, and fungi.

In fact, the cells responsible for fighting infection and foreign invaders in the body (your white blood cells) make hydrogen peroxide and use it to oxidize any offending culprits. The intense bubbling you see when hydrogen peroxide comes in contact with a bacteria-laden cut or wound is the oxygen being released and bacteria being destroyed. The ability of our cells to produce hydrogen peroxide is essential for life. FG-H2O2 is not some undesirable by-product or toxin, but instead a basic requirement for good health.

Newer research indicates we need hydrogen peroxide for a multitude of other chemical reactions that take place throughout the body.

For example, we now know that vitamin C helps fight infections by producing hydrogen peroxide, which in turn stimulates the production of prostaglandins.
Also lactobacillus found in the colon and vagina produce hydrogen peroxide. This destroys harmful bacteria and viruses, preventing colon disease, vaginitis, bladder infections and a host of other common ailments. (Infect Dis News Aug.8,91:5).

When lactobacillus in the colon or vaginal tract have been overrun with harmful viruses, yeast, or bacteria, an effective douche or enema solution can be made using 3 tablespoons of 3% FG-H2O2 in 1 quart of distilled water. Keep in mind, however, that a good bacterial flora must always be re-established in theses areas to achieve lasting results.

While we are discussing enemas and douches, there is another misconception about FG-H2O2 I need to address. The friendly bacteria in the colon and vagina are aerobic. In other words, they flourish in high oxygen environments and thrive in the presence of oxygen rich FG-H2O2.

On the other hand, most strains of harmful bacteria (and cancer cells) are anaerobic and cannot survive in the presence of oxygen or FG-H2O2.

Hydrogen peroxide is safe, readily available and dirt cheap. And best of all, it works!

No one yet fully understands the complete workings of hydrogen peroxide. We do know that it is loaded with oxygen. (A pint of the food-grade 35% solution contains the equivalent of 130 pints of oxygen.

A pint of 3% hydrogen peroxide found at the local drugstore contains 10 pints of oxygen (**although it also has a high degree of solvents, which food grade does not**). And a pint of the 6% solution used to bleach hair contains 20 pints of oxygen.) We also know that when FG-H2O2 is taken into the body (orally or intravenously) the oxygen content of the blood and body tissues increases dramatically.

We are just beginning to learn exactly how FG-H2O2 works. It was reported to work as far back as 1920. The English medical journal, Lancet, then reported that intravenous infusion was used successfully to treat pneumonia in the epidemic following World War I. In the 1940's Father Richard Willhelm, the pioneer in promoting peroxide use, reported on the compound being used extensively to treat everything from bacterial-related mental illness to skin disease and polio.

Father Willhelm is the founder of "Educational Concern for Hydrogen Peroxide" (ECHO, a nonprofit organization dedicated to educating the public on the safe use and therapeutic benefits of hydrogen peroxide.) Much of the interest in hydrogen peroxide waned in the 1940's when prescription medications came on the scene. Since that time there has been little economic interest in funding peroxide research. After all, it is dirt cheap and non-patentable.

Even still, in the last 25 years, over 7,700 articles relating to hydrogen peroxide have been written in the standard medical journals. Thousands more, involving its therapeutic use, have appeared in alternative health publications. The number of conditions helped by hydrogen peroxide is astounding. The reported dangers and side effects are few and often conflicting.

Let's look at several conditions that seem to respond especially well to FG-H2O2 therapy. First, keep in mind that there are two methods of administering the peroxide-orally and intravenously. While most conditions respond remarkably to oral ingestion, emphysema is one condition in which intravenous infusion can be a godsend.

Emphysema involves destruction of the alveoli (the small air sacs in the lungs). Although chemical fumes and other irritants can cause the destruction, it is most often the result of smoking. As the disease progresses, the patient finds it more and more difficult to breathe.

A wheel chair and supplemental oxygen become necessary as the disease progresses. Lack of adequate oxygen reaching the tissues forces the heart to pump more forcefully. This leads to high blood pressure, enlargement of the heart itself and eventually heart failure.

Conventional medicine offers little help for emphysema. There is no cure. The best that can be hoped for is symptomatic relief and the prevention of any serious complications that might result in death. FG-H2O2 therapy can offer more.

Using 1 ounce of 35% peroxide per 1 gallon of non-chlorinated water in a vaporizer improves nighttime breathing tremendously. But intravenous infusion holds the real key to relief. It has the ability to cleanse the inner lining of the lungs and restore the ability to breathe.

With increased pollution it is reacting with airborne toxins before it even reaches the ground.) And everyone, by now, knows the oxygen-generating rain forests are being destroyed worldwide, which further reduces available oxygen. Internal oxygen availability is also under attack.

Chlorination of drinking water removes oxygen. Cooking and over-processing of our foods lowers their oxygen content. Unrestrained antibiotic use destroys beneficial oxygen-creating bacteria in the intestinal tract.

Dr. Johanna Budwig of Germany has shown that for proper cellular utilization of oxygen to take place, our diets must contain adequate amounts of unsaturated fatty acids.

Unfortunately, the oils rich in these fatty acids have become less and less popular with the food industry.

Their very nature makes them more biologically active, which requires more careful processing and gives them a shorter shelf-life. Rather than deal with these challenges, the food industry has turned to the use of synthetic fats and dangerous processes like hydrogenation.

It's obvious that our oxygen needs are not being met. Several of the most common ailments now affecting our population are directly related to oxygen starvation. Asthma, emphysema, and lung disease are on the rise, especially in the polluted metropolitan areas.

Cases of constipation, diarrhea, intestinal parasites and bowel cancer are all on the upswing. Periodontal disease is endemic in the adult population of this country. Cancer of all forms continues to increase. Immune system disorders are sweeping the globe. Chronic fatigue, "Yuppie Flu" and hundreds of other strange viral diseases have begun to surface.

Ironically, many of the new "miracle" drugs and nutritional supplements used to treat these conditions work by increasing cellular oxygen (oftentimes through FG-H2O2 formation). For example, the miracle nutrient, Coenzyme Q10, helps regulate intercellular oxidation.

Organic germanium, which received considerable publicity not too long ago, also increases oxygen levels at the cellular level. And even substances like niacin and vitamin E promote tissue oxidation through their dilation of blood vessels.

Hydrogen peroxide is only one of the many components that help regulate the amount of oxygen getting to your cells. Its presence is vital for many other functions as well.

The closer you look at hydrogen peroxide, the less surprising it becomes that it can help such a wide variety of conditions.

The following is only a partial listing of conditions in which FG-H2O2 therapy has been used successfully. (Many of these conditions are serious, if not life-threatening. As always, I would highly recommend seeking the advice and guidance of a doctor experienced in the use of these techniques.)

Allergies Headaches
Altitude Sickness Herpes Simplex
Alzheimer's Herpes Zoster
Anemia HIV Infection
Arrhythmia Influenza Asthma Insect Bites
Bacterial Infections Liver Cirrhosis
Bronchitis Lupus Erythematosis
Cancer Multiple Sclerosis
Candida Parasitic Infections
Cardiovascular Disease Parkinsonism

Cerebral Vascular Disease Periodontal Disease
Chronic Pain Prostatitis
Diabetes Type 11 Rheumatoid Arthritis
Diabetic Gangrene Shingles
Diabetic Retinopahty Sinusitis
Digestion Problems Sore Throat
Epstein-Barr Infection Ulcers
Emphysema Viral Infections
Food Allergies Warts
Fungal Infections Yeast Infections
Gingivitis

GRADES OF HYDROGEN PEROXIDE (Hydrogen peroxide is available in various strengths and grades).

3% Pharmaceutical Grade: This is the grade sold at your local drugstore or supermarket. This product is not recommended for internal use. It contains an assortment of stabilizers, which shouldn't be ingested. Various stabilizers include: acetanilide, phenol, sodium stanate and tertrasodium phosphate. Additionally, it has a high degree of solvents.

6% Beautician Grade: This is used in beauty shops to color hair and is not recommended for internal use.

30% Reagent Grade: This is used for scientific experimentation and also contains stabilizers. It is also not for internal use.

30% to 32% Electronic Grade: This is used to clean electronic parts and not for internal use.

35% Technical Grade: This is a more concentrated product than the Reagent Grade and differs slightly in that phosphorus is added to help neutralize any chlorine from the water used to dilute it.

35% Food Grade: This is used in the production of foods like cheese, eggs, and whey-containing products. It is also sprayed on the foil lining of aseptic packages containing fruit juices and milk products. **THIS IS THE ONLY GRADE RECOMMENDED FOR INTERNAL USE...**
90%: This is used as an oxygen source for rocket fuel.

Only 35% Food Grade hydrogen peroxide is recommended for internal use. At this concentration, however, hydrogen peroxide is a very strong oxidizer and if not diluted, it can be extremely dangerous or even fatal. Any concentrations over 10% can cause neurological reactions and damage to the upper gastrointestinal tract.

35% Food Grade FG-H2O2 must be 1) handled carefully (direct contact will burn the skin--immediate flushing with water is recommended). 2) diluted properly before use. 3) stored safely and properly (after making a dilution the remainder should be stored tightly sealed in the freezer).

One of the most convenient methods of dispensing 35% FG-H2O2 is from a small glass eye dropper bottle. These can be purchased at your local drugstore. Fill this with the 35% FG-H_2O_2 and store the larger container in the freezer compartment of your refrigerator until more is needed. Store the eye dropper bottle in the refrigerator.

FLOURIDE

Fluoride: Wide Range of Serious Health Problems

Respected Medical Professionals and Scientists are warning that water fluoridation has dangerous long-term consequences to health. For over 50 years, the U.S. government and media have trumpeted fluoride as a safe and effective means of reducing cavities, especially in children. But fluoride is not the benevolent and innocuous substance the public has been led to believe.

Fluoride is a corrosive poison that will produce serious effects on a long range basis. Any attempt to use water this way is deplorable." Dr. Charles Gordon Heyd, Past President of the American Medical Association.

Dr Robert Verkerk - "Fluorides are extremely reactive molecules which have been shown to cause considerable harm in biological systems. They continue to be used by health authorities for a specific medicinal purpose, namely the treatment and prevention of dental caries, yet they have never been subjected to the full risk/benefit analysis which is required in order to bring other drugs to the market.

Drinking water medicated with fluoride clearly amounts to government-sponsored use of an unlicenced drug. It is staggering that international bodies such as the United Nations' Codex Alimentarius Commission could have overruled the substantial scientific concerns about fluoride in infant formula raised by several countries in November's Codex meeting in Chiang Mai, Thailand and that babies, the most vulnerable members of our society, are made the innocent victims." Dr Robert Verkerk, Executive Director of the Alliance for Natural Health.

August 2002 - Belgium becomes the first country in the world to prohibit fluoride supplements Fluoride tablets, fluoride drops and fluoride chewing gum, for decades promoted as the crown jewels of dentistry, are going to be taken off the market because they are poisonous and pose a great risk for physical and psychological health. This has been decided by the Federal Minister of Public Health.

"Fluoridation ... it is the greatest fraud that has ever been perpetrated and it has been perpetrated on more people than any other fraud has."Professor Albert Schatz, Ph.D. (Microbiology), Discoverer of streptomycin and Nobel Prize Winner.

14th Nov 2005 - Most of Western Europe has now abandoned fluoridation of water due to a lack of evidence as to its effectiveness and concerns about major side-effects. 98% of Europe is now free of fluoridated water.

EMERGENCY, SURVIVAL & FIRST AID PREPARATION

Some Ways to Prepare for the Absolute Worst
You don't have to go as far as a survivalist, but you can certainly learn from them. Here is a distillation of advice from emergency preparedness experts from across the spectrum:

WATER

If you take nothing else away from this article, at least heed this advice: stock up on water. It is cheap, it has a long shelf-life, and, most important, you cannot live without it. Most of us can do without food - not to mention e-mail - for several weeks.

But dehydration is a very real and life-threatening danger after a calamity. Though you drink half a gallon of water a day, you should store one gallon of water per person per day. Assume you will be cut off for at least three days and store as much extra as you have room for in a cool, dark space. The International Bottled Water Association says jugs of water can be kept indefinitely, though they may pick up an off-flavor from the plastic after a year or so. But it is pretty easy to rotate the stock every

couple of months since many people drink bottled water.
If you have the room, store some of the water in the freezer. When the electricity goes, you'll have more ice to preserve the food in the refrigerator for a day or two longer.

If worse comes to worse and you run out of water while your community's water supply is contaminated, turn off the water supply to your house and drain water from your water heater or scoop it from the toilet tank. It must be purified by boiling it for several minutes or by mixing in two drops of old-fashioned bleach - not the "mountain fresh" scented varieties - to each quart of water.

FOOD

The odds of anything calamitous happening are slim, so you don't want to spend several thousand dollars buying and storing food. You have better things to do with your money than investing in creamed corn and sardines. If you have a pantry or basement with a decent supply of canned foods and bottled juices, you should do just fine for several weeks. "You could survive for two weeks just on Tang," said Eric Zaltas, nutritionist with PowerBar Inc., a maker of nutrition bars.

Given that in most emergencies - floods, earthquake or fire - you may have to flee, it is smart to keep a 72-hour bug-out kit. That's a three-day supply that you can easily carry out

to the car at a moment's notice. The crucial concept here is high nutrition in a small amount of space. Freeze-dried foods would be perfect, except you'll need clean and heated water to reconstitute those products.
Some people buy the military's Meals Ready to Eat (MRE's). A case of 12 meals costs about $73 and they are currently in short supply. Nutrition bars are another good choice. The rap against them - loads of fat, carbohydrates and calories - is actually a plus during a disaster. Something like the PowerBar Performance Bar also contains electrolytes, which when taken with water, will help keep your body chemistry in order. Avoid the chocolate-coated varieties because they will just get messy when it gets hot and water for cleanup is at a premium.

High-protein diet shakes are a bit expensive, but have the added advantage of supplying you with liquid, as would high-fiber potassium-packed vegetable juice. Throw in some dried fruit and you have enough calories to get by for three days.
Don't forget ready-to-feed baby formula if you have an infant. People with medical conditions like diabetes or kidney disease will have to pay more attention to what they store and what they eat.

CASH

If you get a warning, head to the nearest cash machine ASAP. (You'll already have all the food and water you need, right?) The time to raid the

A.T.M. is before the disaster because when the electricity fails, you won't find one that works. Take out as much as you can because you may need it to buy supplies at post-disaster inflated prices and credit cards won't work if there is no electricity or computer networks are down. When the disaster has passed put the money back in the bank.

COMMUNICATIONS

In almost every disaster, cellphones have proved remarkably useless. (Old-fashioned landline phones hold up much better.) Without electricity, desktop computers become expensive paperweights and laptops follow in short order as their batteries drain. Short of a $1,000 satellite phone, there is precious little you can do to reach out to the world in an emergency.

Two things that might help: get an e-mail account from Google or Yahoo that allows you access to e-mail from any computer you happen to find and buy a hand-crank cell phone charger.

EXTRAS

You cannot do without a first-aid kit, a radio and lots of batteries. The new flashlights that use light-emitting diodes will help you conserve juice. Camping gear - butane stoves, coolers and lightweight tents - easily doubles as survival gear. What else? An adapter that turns your car's cigarette lighter into an electrical outlet for any appliance could be a lifesaver. Consider sticking a can of fluorescent spray paint among your other supplies and then stash all this stuff in a plastic box that can serve to float things out to safety.

MEDICINES

Thanks to health insurance companies' rules, it is often not easy to get extra medicine without paying full price. But with a little planning it can be done. Or for several months in a row, start refilling prescriptions a week or so before they run out until you have accumulated several weeks' supply.

DOCUMENTS

Pulling together documents you need on the run may be the hardest thing to do. Financial planners have been after people for years to make a "beneficiary book" to help their heirs or executors more easily sort through affairs. It should hold copies of birth and marriage certificates, adoption papers, key identification numbers, copies of bank statements, deeds, titles, credit cards and insurance policies as well as passwords to online accounts. The same information would be useful to you in case you lose access to your primary records in a disaster. Just keep it in a secure place and grab it on the way out of the house.
Where to shop and Stock
Food, water & supplies

HORMONE REPLACEMENT THERAPY (HRT)

In today's society women are conditioned to think that it is a natural occurrence to experience menopause. Many have accepted it as something God has put in place for every woman once she has reached a certain age. However, it has been proven by many schools of thought that you are what you eat. Sarah, Abraham's wife conceived a child at the age of ninety years old. Even though God blessed her, she had to be preserved and strong enough to withstand the burden of carrying a child, especially considering what a ninety-year old woman look like today. What kind of food was she eating? Was it the same food that women of this generation eat? Did they have organic food in those days? What about solvents, toxins and parasites? What about drinking alcohol and smoking cigarettes? Did she eat a lot of sugar, starches, fruits and vegetables? The point is, was Sarah made of the same material the women of today are made of, or is it the food that made her different?

According to Messenger Elijah Muhammad, alcohol and tobacco has a poisonous effect upon the body; it cuts the life span down, as far as reproductive organs are concerned. And nowadays, with dope added to all of the above - mentioned poisonous food and drinks, we can easily say with truth, that the people are committing suicide. As a result of the continual use of this poison, they lose sexual desires at an early age. Tobacco and whiskey will most certainly destroy it. The flesh of swine and alcoholic drinks will give a false impression of feeling to the victim. As if they can do things that they can't. These things are death to children in their early ages, because not only does it affect their reproductive system, but also the heart, lungs, and sharpness of thinking. And, after all of this, you die a victim of poison and commercialization.

According to Dr. Hulda Clark, as a result of the food being polluted with solvents and parasites, the body cannot purify it self properly. She went on to say that no menopausal symptoms are normal. After the ovaries are done with their cycles of estrogen and progesterone production, the adrenal glands' hormone production was meant to kick in and make up for the deficiency. They should be able to keep your hormone levels regulated.

Natural Progesterone

Since the total truth came out about HRT, the medical community has been in turmoil and somewhat divided as to what should be recommended to women who are experiencing symptoms of hormonal imbalance. In the meantime millions of women are confused about what to do to relieve their symptoms and at the same time not cause health problems down the road.

Natural progesterone cream, when used correctly, seems to help many women through the symptoms of hormonal imbalance with many added benefits. Natural progesterone, has the same molecular structure as the progesterone produced by the body. It is absorbed through the skin and into the bloodstream. It can help your body keep estrogen and progesterone levels in balance, resulting in maintained sense of equilibrium.

As beneficial as natural progesterone cream is, we must be aware that we are dealing with a very delicate system - the endocrine system. According to Dr. Joseph Mercola: "The problem relates to the fact that progesterone is highly fat soluble and once applied to the skin will store itself in a woman's fat tissue. When one first uses the cream, there is no problem here as the fat stores are very low. But as time goes on, the cream accumulates and contributes to disruptions in the adrenal hormones such as DHEA, cortisol, and testosterone. Although progesterone cream is an enormously useful tool, it should be used very cautiously.

It is advised that women test their progesterone levels yearly. Although progesterone over-dose is not something that causes great harm, initially-sleepiness is a clue-the solution that we are after is balance of all hormones. Anytime there is an over-balance of a hormone, even progesterone, the system will suffer and symptoms will appear.

Along with progesterone, balancing the adrenals is very important, but something that is often over-looked in hormonal balancing. There are many useful herbs that can help accomplish this along with the following: Diet, Stress and Sleep.
A totally balanced diet, is very important. Most hormonal symptoms can be relieved with a healthy, balanced diet. Along with diet, drinking plenty pure water.

Hidden stress can be the underlying cause of why some women do not experience symptom relief of hormonal imbalance. Stress is often a "silent symptom" in that we have usually learned to consider it as being a normal part of life. Some suggestions in dealing with stress include: meditation, prayer, yoga, EFT, exercise (especially walking), deep breathing and learning how to remove yourself from difficult situations. In order to alleviate stress these must be practiced very daily.

It is said that over ¾ of the population is sleep deprived. The importance of being in bed before 10:00 p.m. so that the body's biorhythms will react every night at the same time. The body does most of its repair and healing between the hours of 10:00 p.m. and 2:00 a.m. If you are awake during these hours your body definitely looses. There is no such thing as "catching up on your sleep". Once it is lost, it cannot be regained.

Like most things in life, we must always proceed with caution. There is no magic bullet when it comes to getting the body balanced and healthy. Natural progesterone is the most natural and safest way to assist women with the symptoms of hormonal imbalance, but we must remember that our goal is "balance" in every area.

The following table shows the benefits of natural progesterone compared to estrogen. As you can see, the effects of progesterone are many-we would do well to use it wisely.

Estrogen Effects:

Stimulates breasts cysts; Increases body fat storage; Salt and fluid retention; Depression and headaches; Interferes with thyroid hormone; Increases blood clotting and risk of stroke; Decreases libido (sex drive);

Too much estrogen (estrogen dominance) causes the body to become less sensitive to thyroid hormone. In other words, you will have normal or low thyroid hormone by lab test, but look hypothyroid. Thus, too much estrogen causes hypothyroid even though lab tests are normal. If you are hypothyroid due to estrogen dominance, then you will have fat on the hips and thinning hair. Natural Progesterone will reverse too much estrogen and oppose estrogen, IF you avoid xenoestrogens. Thus, it may become easier to lose fat on the belly and hips and grow thicker hair when you take Natural Progesterone and have normal thyroid function.

The list of foods below contain natural estrogen and estrogen inhibiting properties. The foods we need to sustain life comes completely equipt with all the vitamins and minerals we need. It is wise to be aware to prevent over indulgence by practicing moderation.

Alfalfa
Animal flesh
Anise seed
Apples
Baker's yeast
Barley
Beets
Carrots
Cherries
Chickpeas
Clover
Cucumbers
Dairy Foods
Dates
Eggs
Eggplant
Fennel
Flaxseeds
Garlic
Hops
Licorice
Oats
Olive oil
Olives

Papaya
Parsley
Peas
Peppers
Plums
Pomegranates
Potatoes
Pumpkin
Red beans
Red clover
Rhubarb
Rice
Sage
Sesame seeds
Soybean sprouts
Soybeans
Split peas
Sunflower seeds
Tomatoes
Wheat
Yams

Estrogen Inhibiting Foods:

If you are suffering from breast cancer, PMS, fibroids, ovarian cysts, and other situations that estrogen might exacerbate, the following estrogen inhibiting foods might be of interest to you.

Berries
Broccoli
Cabbage
Citrus Foods
Corn
Figs

Fruits (except apples, cherries, dates, pomegranates)
Grapes
Green beans
Melons
Millet
Onions
Pears
Pineapples
Squashes
Tapioca

Natural Progesterone is known as the "happy hormone". During the third trimester of pregnancy, the placenta produces 400 mg/day of Natural Progesterone (20 times the normal dose). After delivery (the placenta is delivered too), progesterone drops to zero and then you get post partum depression.

Impairs blood sugar control; Loss of zinc and retention of copper; Reduced oxygen level in all cells; Increased risk of endometrial cancer; Increased risk of breast cancer; Helps decrease bone loss slightly.
Progesterone Effects: Protects against breast cysts; Helps use fat for energy and keep it off hips; Natural diuretic (water pill); Natural anti-depressant; Facilitates thyroid hormone action; Normalizes blood clotting; Increases libido; Normalizes blood sugar levels; Normalizes zinc and copper levels; Restores proper cell oxygen levels; Prevents endometrial cancer; Helps prevent breast cancer; Increases bone building.

CAN MEN USE PROGESTERONE?

Males make progesterone. They need it to make their testosterone and for the adrenal glands to make cortisone. Males synthesize progesterone in amounts less than women do but it is still vital. You can measure male's progesterone levels, and you'll find that when the woman has this follicle damage, the amount of progesterone she makes is less than that of a male.

Men with BPH (swelling of the prostate) and other male related problems will appreciate the speed of relief with progesterone cream. Dr. Lee recommends that men use 8 - 12 mg of progesterone daily. Progesterone has NO feminizing characteristics. Progesterone is a 5-alpha reductase inhibitor -- it helps prevent the conversion of testosterone into DHT.

(John R. Lee, M.D. was internationally acknowledged as a pioneer and expert in the study and use of the hormone progesterone, and on the subject of hormone replacement therapy for women. He used transdermal progesterone extensively in his clinical practice for nearly a decade, doing research which showed that it can reverse osteoporosis. Dr. Lee also famously coined the term "estrogen dominance," meaning a relative lack of progesterone compared to estrogen, which causes a list of symptoms familiar to millions of women.)

Progesterone may also help men with complexion and increased energy. Progesterone balances the estrogens that build in a man's body. Furthermore, it may be important in the prevention and/or treatment of prostatism and prostate cancer. Dr Lee has had men contact him telling him that as a result of applying progesterone cream to their wife they were seeing that their symptoms of prostatism such as urinary urgency and frequency decreased considerably. Several men with prostate cancer reported that their PSA (Prostate Specific Antigen) level decreased and they have had no progression of their prostate lesions since using the cream themselves. Another man contacted Dr Lee to say his bone metastases are now no longer visible by Mayo Clinic X-ray tests. After reviewing endocrinology books in regard to hormone changes in older men Dr Lee found that progesterone levels drop, estradiol levels rise, and testosterone changes in form in older men. This is significant enough to warrant research to determine if the application of progesterone can be used to prevent prostrate cancer.

Closing remarks: According to the above information, it is obvious that there is no differentiating between male and female when it comes to imbalances. Once the organs are deficient in something, they are going to react.

The body should be fed properly like an organic plant. If you organically nourish it with the best natural foods without chemicals or pesticides, the more holistic and power packed with vitamins and mineral it will be. It will bear new fruit over and over again before it dies. But initially when it is eaten, the body will get the benefit of a natural food that is being distributed proportionately through out the body in the different areas that need it most. This in itself is a protection to all the organs because they are being nourished with the proper food and not clogged with unnatural things that shouldn't be there. Therefore they can keep the body balanced and in check. However, if it is not allowed to grow the way it was created, naturally without the aide of chemicals and pollutants, it will product an unnatural product that the body may not recognize; thereby, creating imbalances and other problems.

Unfortunately, when there is an imbalance, it can throw the system completely off and it can takes a long time to re-group. It may depend on how long it has been deficient. That is where the help of certain hormonal balancing products may help such as progesterone. There are many progesterone creams with which many people have had progress and they come highly recommended.

For more information see sources in back of book.

WEIGHT and OVER- EATING PROBLEMS

Is It a psychological way of finding balance ?

The most common element surrounding ALL Eating Disorders is the inherent presence of a low self – esteem

Compulsive Overeating:

People suffering with Compulsive Overeating have what is characterized as an "addiction" to food, using food and eating as a way to hide from their emotions, to fill a void they feel inside, and to cope with daily stresses and problems in their lives.

People suffering with this Eating Disorder tend to be overweight, are usually aware that their eating habits are abnormal, but find little comfort because of society's tendency to stereotype the "overweight" individual. Words like, "just go on a diet" are as emotionally devastating to a person suffering Compulsive Overeating as "just eat" can be to a person suffering Anorexia. A person suffering as a Compulsive Overeater is at health risk for a heart attack, high blood-pressure and cholesterol, kidney disease and/or failure, arthritis and bone deterioration, and stroke.

Men and Women who are Compulsive Overeaters will sometimes hide behind their physical appearance, using it as a blockade against society (common in survivors of sexual abuse). They feel guilty for not being "good enough," shame for being overweight, and generally have a very low self-esteem... they use food and eating to cope with these feelings, which only leads into the cycle of feeling them ten-fold and trying to find a way to cope again. With a low self esteem and often constant need

for love and validation he/she will turn to obsessive episodes of binging and eating as a way to forget the pain and the desire for affection.
It is important to remember that most Eating Disorders, though their signs and symptoms may be different, share a great number of common causes and emotional aspects.

The Honorable Elijah Muhammad teaches to use moderation when it comes to the diet. He has stated on many occasions, that food can prolong life or shorten life if it is not the right kind of food and eaten at the proper time.

In today's society food is one of the best advertising tools around. If you have a weight problem, it is almost impossible to diet, especially if you're a couch potato (watch a lot of TV). Yet, it is possible to control one's weight if it is done in stages. Instead of a sudden drastic approach of dropping all to your favorite foods at once, start by cutting back on portions, then cut back on snacks and in -between meals. Then cut back on the number of meals you eat per day as indicated in How to Eat to Live. The results will be very rewarding if you can take the first step at taking control of your life back. You owe it to yourself. Over eating can cause many health problems, even death. Eat to live, not to die.

DOCTORS, SICKNESS & HEALTH

Interestingly Messenger Elijah Muhammad points out throughout his books that considering the limited existence the Caucasians have been on our planet, they are constantly experimenting on the peoples of the earth. They are given credit for their discoveries and inventive natures, but at what cost? The world is becoming more polluted the more they experiment. Yet, how many more lives must be lost in the process?

The medical industry and its doctors have paid large sums of money to attend school and are hard pressed to pay back great loans and maintain expensive lifestyles. They become bound to it and have to charge you great sums of money. It likewise ties into perpetuating the system of advising the people to eat "normally," which in affect will keep them coming to the doctors, because there is no cure in medicine. The doctors doesn't promote cure; they promote relieving the symptoms with medicine or cutting it off or out. This still leaves you vulnerable to them and the pharmaceutical industry taking pills the rest of your life.

One thing that stands out however, the doctors are victim to the same sickness they treat their patients for. This shows us that they don't know as much as we have been made to think they do.

This book is not suggesting that they know nothing. In some cases medicine or surgery may be necessary, but in last resorts. If the people were taught to eat properly at infancy, their fragile organs will be built properly and would be able to withstand the strain when of age; however, we tend to taught to eat three or more meals a day wearing our tender stomach lining out before they ever form strength. Infants are given hog and every other type of meat, knowing they have no teeth to help in the process of breaking it down; consequently, that meat sits in their fragile stomachs forcing all of its digestive juices to work on it and it still doesn't do a good job. This make the whole system work tremendously hard to process such heavy and difficultly digestive food.

Add to this chemicalization of formula, milk, juices, and the like, the kidneys and liver are taxed as well. It is no wonder kidney and liver failure are so rampant today due to these purifying organs being worked beyond their capacity before they are even formed well. We are then in the long line for dialysis treatment, because our kidneys stop functioning. As usual, the doctor is advising us once again on how to maintain our appointments.

We believe that there is no compulsion is what we or God offers. The doctors have made it clear from hundreds of years of trial and error that a little knowledge is dangerous. Why not try God and the natural processes for our natural bodies? He is the Best Knower.

He teaches that by eating one meal a day minimally, at the same time, trains our stomachs to call for food only then. He also teaches us that we should only eat when we are hungry. It is resting of the digestive track which is the key to long life and eating the proper good food at the same time daily that will prolong our lives. The reader and practitioner of this principle will have more life abundantly as promised by Allah (God), Who came in the person of Master Fard Muhammad, given to us from His Last and Greatest Messenger, Elijah Muhammad.

RESOURCES, CONTACTS & RECOMMENDED SITES

Product	Site Links
Books	Overstock.com
	indiaclub.com
Herbs, Teas, Spices	herbalremedies.com
	glenbrookfarm.com
Internal Cleansing Kits	blessedherbs.com
	Qnlabs.com
Dishwashing Detergent	ecoproducts.com
	soapsgonebuy.com
Glass Cookware	cooking.com
	tabletools.com
Natural Cosmetics	naturalcosmetics.com
	purebodysolutions.com
Cosmetics-Men of Color	skincare.com
Survival Kits	quakekare.com
	preparedness.com
Progesterone	natural-progesterone-advisory-network.com
	conceivingconcepts.com
Juicer	jr.com

Sugar in the raw	minimus.biz
Kosher Cheese	
Kosher grocery store	kosher.com
Alta Dena cheese	careerbuilder.com
Appliances	ekitchengadgets.com
Whole Food Supplements	qnlabs.com
Water Filter	ecoviva.com
	Ewater.com
Alternative Medicine	vitacost.com
	herbalremedies.com
Peroxide (Food Grade	rawfood.com
Toothpaste	ecoviva.com
	vitacost.com
Shea Butter	theafricanstore.org
	alaffia.com
	oilsbynature.com

GLOSSARY OF TERMS

This list of animal ingredients and their alternatives helps consumers avoid animal ingredients in food, cosmetics, and other products. Please note, however, that it is not all-inclusive. There are thousands of technical and patented names for ingredient variations. Furthermore, many ingredients known by one name can be of animal, vegetable, or synthetic origin. If you have a question regarding an ingredient in a product, call the manufacturer. Good sources of additional information are the Consumer's Dictionary of Cosmetic Ingredients, the Consumer's Dictionary of Food Additives, or an unabridged dictionary.

All of these are available at most libraries:

A

Adrenaline.
Hormone from adrenal glands of hogs, cattle, and sheep. In medicine. Alternatives: synthetics.

Alanine.
(See Amino Acids.)

Albumen.
In eggs, milk, muscles, blood, and many vegetable tissues and fluids. In cosmetics,

albumen is usually derived from egg whites and used as a coagulating agent. May cause allergic reaction. In cakes, cookies, candies, etc. Egg whites sometimes used in "clearing" wines. Derivative: Albumin.

Albumin.
(See Albumen.)

Alcloxa.
(See Allantoin.)

Aldioxa.
(See Allantoin.)

Aliphatic Alcohol.
(See Lanolin and Vitamin A.)

Allantoin.
Uric acid from cows, most mammals. Also in many plants (especially comfrey). In cosmetics (especially creams and lotions) and used in treatment of wounds and ulcers. Derivatives: Alcloxa, Aldioxa. Alternatives: extract of comfrey root, synthetics.

Alligator Skin.
(See Leather.)

Alpha-Hydroxy Acids.
Any one of several acids used as an exfoliant and in anti-wrinkle products. Lactic acid may be animal-derived (see Lactic Acid). Alternatives: glycolic acid, citric acid, and salicylic acid are plant- or fruit-derived.

Ambergris.
From whale intestines. Used as a fixative in making perfumes and as a flavoring in foods and beverages. Alternatives: synthetic or vegetable fixatives.

Amino Acids.
The building blocks of protein in all animals and plants. In cosmetics, vitamins, supplements, shampoos, etc. Alternatives: synthetics, plant sources.

Aminosuccinate Acid.
(See Aspartic Acid.)

Angora.
Hair from the Angora rabbit or goat. Used in clothing. Alternatives: synthetic fibers.

Animal Fats and Oils.
In foods, cosmetics, etc. Highly allergenic. Alternatives: olive oil, wheat germ oil, coconut oil, flaxseed oil, almond oil, safflower oil, etc.

Animal Hair.
In some blankets, mattresses, brushes, furniture, etc. Alternatives: vegetable and synthetic fibers.

Arachidonic Acid.
A liquid unsaturated fatty acid that is found in liver, brain, glands, and fat of animals and humans. Generally isolated from animal liver. Used in companion animal food for nutrition and in skin creams and lotions to soothe

eczema and rashes. Alternatives: synthetics, aloe vera, tea tree oil, calendula ointment.

Arachidyl Proprionate.
A wax that can be from animal fat. Alternatives: peanut or vegetable oil.

Aspartic Acid. Aminosuccinate Acid.
Can be animal or plant source (e.g., molasses). Sometimes synthesized for commercial purposes.

B

Bee Pollen.
Microsporic grains in seed plants gathered by bees then collected from the legs of bees. Causes allergic reactions in some people. In nutritional supplements, shampoos, toothpastes, deodorants. Alternatives: synthetics, plant amino acids, pollen collected from plants.

Bee Products.
Produced by bees for their own use. Bees are selectively bred. Culled bees are killed. A cheap sugar is substituted for their stolen honey. Millions die as a result. Their legs are often torn off by pollen-collection trapdoors.

Beeswax. Honeycomb.
Wax obtained from melting honeycomb with boiling water, straining it, and cooling it. From virgin bees. Very cheap and widely used but

harmful to the skin. In lipsticks and many other cosmetics (especially face creams, lotions, mascara, eye creams and shadows, face makeups, nail whiteners, lip balms, etc.). Derivatives: Cera Flava. Alternatives: paraffin, vegetable oils and fats. Ceresin aka ceresine aka earth wax. (Made from the mineral ozokerite. Replaces beeswax in cosmetics. Also used to wax paper, to make polishing cloths, in dentistry for taking wax impressions, and in candle-making.) Also, carnauba wax (from the Brazilian palm tree; used in many cosmetics, including lipstick; rarely causes allergic reactions). Candelilla wax (from candelilla plants; used in many cosmetics, including lipstick; also in the manufacture of rubber, phonograph records, in waterproofing and writing inks; no known toxicity). Japan wax (Vegetable wax. Japan tallow. Fat from the fruit of a tree grown in Japan and China.).

Benzoic Acid.
In almost all vertebrates and in berries. Used as a preservative in mouthwashes, deodorants, creams, aftershave lotions, etc. Alternatives: cranberries, gum benzoin (tincture) from the aromatic balsamic resin from trees grown in China, Sumatra, Thailand, and Cambodia.

Beta Carotene.
(See Carotene.)

Biotin. Vitamin H. Vitamin B Factor.
In every living cell and in larger amounts in milk and yeast. Used as a texturizer in

cosmetics, shampoos, and creams. Alternatives: plant sources.

Blood.
From any slaughtered animal. Used as adhesive in plywood, also found in cheese-making, foam rubber, intravenous feedings, and medicines. Possibly in foods such as lecithin. Alternatives: synthetics, plant sources.
Boar Bristles.
Hair from wild or captive hogs. In "natural" toothbrushes and bath and shaving brushes. Alternatives: vegetable fibers, nylon, the peelu branch or peelu gum (Asian, available in the U.S., its juice replaces toothpaste).

Bone Char.
Animal bone ash. Used in bone china and often to make sugar white. Serves as the charcoal used in aquarium filters. Alternatives: synthetic tribasic calcium phosphate.

Bone Meal.
Crushed or ground animal bones. In some fertilizers. In some vitamins and supplements as a source of calcium. In toothpastes. Alternatives: plant mulch, vegetable compost, dolomite, clay, vegetarian vitamins.

C
Calciferol.
(See Vitamin D.)

Calfskin.
(See Leather.)

Caprylamine Oxide.
(See Caprylic Acid.)

Capryl Betaine.
(See Caprylic Acid.)

Caprylic Acid.
A liquid fatty acid from cow's or goat's milk. Also from palm and coconut oil, other plant oils. In perfumes, soaps. Derivatives: Caprylic Triglyceride, Caprylamine Oxide, Capryl Betaine. Alternatives: plant sources.

Caprylic Triglyceride.
(See Caprylic Acid.)

Carbamide.
(See Urea.)

Carmine. Cochineal. Carminic Acid.
Red pigment from the crushed female cochineal insect. Reportedly 70,000 beetles must be killed to produce one pound of this red dye. Used in cosmetics, shampoos, red apple sauce, and other foods (including red lollipops and food coloring). May cause allergic reaction. Alternatives: beet juice (used in powders, rouges, shampoos; no known toxicity); alkanet root (from the root of this herblike tree; used as a red dye for inks, wines, lip balms, etc.; no known toxicity. Can also be combined to make a copper or blue coloring). (See Colors.)

Carminic Acid.
(See Carmine.)

Carotene. Provitamin A. Beta Carotene.
A pigment found in many animal tissues and in all plants. Used as a coloring in cosmetics and in the manufacture of vitamin A.

Casein. Caseinate. Sodium Caseinate.
Milk protein. In "non-dairy" creamers, soy cheese, many cosmetics, hair preparations, beauty masks. Alternatives: soy protein, soy milk, and other vegetable milks.

Caseinate.
(See Casein.)

Cashmere.
Wool from the Kashmir goat. Used in clothing. Alternatives: synthetic fibers.

Castor. Castoreum.
Creamy substance with strong odor from muskrat and beaver genitals. Used as a fixative in perfume and incense. Alternatives: synthetics, plant castor oil. Castoreum. (See Castor.)

Catgut.
Tough string from the intestines of sheep, horses, etc. Used for surgical sutures. Also for stringing tennis rackets and musical instruments, etc. Alternatives: nylon and other synthetic fibers.

Cera Flava.
(See Beeswax.)

Cetyl Alcohol.
Wax found in spermaceti from sperm whales or dolphins. Alternatives: vegetable cetyl alcohol (e.g., coconut), synthetic spermaceti.

Cetyl Palmitate.
(See Spermaceti.)

Chitosan.
A fiber derived from crustacean shells. Used as a lipid binder in diet products. Alternatives: raspberries, yams, legumes, dried apricots, and many other fruits and vegetables.

Cholesterin.
(See Lanolin.)

Cholesterol.
A steroid alcohol in all animal fats and oils, nervous tissue, egg yolk, and blood. Can be derived from lanolin. In cosmetics, eye creams, shampoos, etc. Alternatives: solid complex alcohols (sterols) from plant sources.

Choline Bitartrate.
(See Lecithin.)

Civet.
Unctuous secretion painfully scraped from a gland very near the genital organs of civet cats. Used as a fixative in perfumes. Alternatives: (See alternatives to Musk).

Cochineal.
(See Carmine.)

Cod Liver Oil.
(See Marine Oil.)

Collagen.
Fibrous protein in vertebrates. Usually derived from animal tissue. Can't affect the skin's own collagen. An allergen. Alternatives: soy protein, almond oil, amla oil (see alternative to Keratin), etc.

Colors. Dyes.
Pigments from animal, plant, and synthetic sources used to color foods, cosmetics, and other products. Cochineal is from insects. Widely used FD&C and D&C colors are coal-tar (bituminous coal) derivatives that are continously tested on animals due to their carcinogenic properties. Alternatives: grapes, beets, turmeric, saffron, carrots, chlorophyll, annatto, alkanet.

Corticosteroid.
(See Cortisone.)

Cortisone. Corticosteroid.
Hormone from adrenal glands. Widely used in medicine. Alternatives: synthetics.

Cysteine, L-Form.
An amino acid from hair which can come from animals. Used in hair-care products and creams, in some bakery products, and in

wound-healing formulations. Alternatives: plant sources.

Cystine.
An amino acid found in urine and horsehair. Used as a nutritional supplement and in emollients. Alternatives: plant sources.

D

Dexpanthenol.
(See Panthenol.)
Diglycerides.
(See Monoglycerides and Glycerin.)

Dimethyl Stearamine.
(See Stearic Acid.)

Down.
Goose or duck insulating feathers. From slaughtered or cruelly exploited geese. Used as an insulator in quilts, parkas, sleeping bags, pillows, etc. Alternatives: polyester and synthetic substitutes, kapok (silky fibers from the seeds of some tropical trees) and milkweed seed pod fibers.

Duodenum Substances.
From the digestive tracts of cows and pigs. Added to some vitamin tablets. In some medicines. Alternatives: vegetarian vitamins, synthetics.

Dyes.

(See Colors.)

E

Egg Protein.
In shampoos, skin preparations, etc. Alternatives: plant proteins.

Elastin.
Protein found in the neck ligaments and aortas of cows. Similar to collagen. Can't affect the skin's own elasticity. Alternatives: synthetics, protein from plant tissues.
Emu Oil.
From flightless ratite birds native to Australia and now factory farmed. Used in cosmetics, creams. Alternatives: vegetable and plant oils.

Ergocalciferol.
(See Vitamin D.)

Ergosterol.
(See Vitamin D.)

Estradiol.
(See Estrogen.)

Estrogen. Estradiol.
Female hormones from pregnant mare's urine. Considered a drug. Can have harmful systemic effects if used by children. Used for reproductive problems and in birth control pills and in Premarin, a menopausal drug. In creams, perfumes, and lotions. Has a negligible effect in

the creams as a skin restorative; simple vegetable-source emollients are considered better. Alternatives: oral contraceptives and menopausal drugs based on synthetic steroids or phytoestrogens (from plants, especially palm-kernel oil). Menopausal symptoms can also be treated with diet and herbs.

F

Fats.
(See Animal Fats.)

Fatty Acids.
Can be one or any mixture of liquid and solid acids such as caprylic, lauric, myristic, oleic, palmitic, and stearic. Used in bubble baths, lipsticks, soap, detergents, cosmetics, food. Alternatives: vegetable-derived acids, soy lecithin, safflower oil, bitter almond oil, sunflower oil, etc.

FD&C Colors.
(See Colors.)

Feathers.
From exploited and slaughtered birds. Used whole as ornaments or ground up in shampoos. (See Down and Keratin.)

Fish Liver Oil.
Used in vitamins and supplements. In milk fortified with vitamin D. Alternatives: yeast

extract ergosterol and exposure of skin to sunshine.

Fish Oil.
(See Marine Oil.) Fish oil can also be from marine mammals. Used in soap-making.

Fish Scales.
Used in shimmery makeups. Alternatives: mica, rayon, synthetic pearl.

Fur.
Obtained from animals (usually mink, foxes, or rabbits) cruelly trapped in steel-jaw leghold traps or raised in intensive confinement on fur "farms." Alternatives: synthetics. (See Sable Brushes.)

G

Gel.
(See Gelatin.)

Gelatin. Gel.
Protein obtained by boiling skin, tendons, ligaments, and/or bones with water. From cows and pigs. Used in shampoos, face masks, and other cosmetics. Used as a thickener for fruit gelatins and puddings (e.g., "Jello"). In candies, marshmallows, cakes, ice cream, yogurts. On photographic film and in vitamins as a coating and as capsules. Sometimes used to assist in "clearing" wines. Alternatives: carrageen (carrageenan, Irish moss), seaweeds (algin,

agar-agar, kelp--used in jellies, plastics, medicine), pectin from fruits, dextrins, locust bean gum, cotton gum, silica gel. Marshmallows were originally made from the root of the marsh mallow plant. Vegetarian capsules are now available from several companies. Digital cameras don't use film.

Glucose Tyrosinase.
(See Tyrosine.)

Glycerides.
(See Glycerin.)

Glycerin. Glycerol.
A byproduct of soap manufacture (normally uses animal fat). In cosmetics, foods, mouthwashes, chewing gum, toothpastes, soaps, ointments, medicines, lubricants, transmission and brake fluid, and plastics. Derivatives: Glycerides, Glyceryls, Glycreth-26, Polyglycerol. Alternatives: vegetable glycerin--a byproduct of vegetable oil soap. Derivatives of seaweed, petroleum.
Glycerol.
(See Glycerin.)

Glyceryls.
(See Glycerin.)

Glycreth-26.
(See Glycerin.)

Guanine. Pearl Essence.

Obtained from scales of fish. Constituent of ribonucleic acid and deoxyribonucleic acid and found in all animal and plant tissues. In shampoo, nail polish, other cosmetics. Alternatives: leguminous plants, synthetic pearl, or aluminum and bronze particles.

H

Hide Glue.
Same as gelatin but of a cruder impure form. Alternatives: dextrins and synthetic petrochemical-based adhesives. (See Gelatin.)

Honey.
Food for bees, made by bees. Can cause allergic reactions. Used as a coloring and an emollient in cosmetics and as a flavoring in foods. Should never be fed to infants. Alternatives: in foods--maple syrup, date sugar, syrups made from grains such as barley malt, turbinado sugar, molasses; in cosmetics--vegetable colors and oils.

Honeycomb.
(See Beeswax.)
Horsehair.
(See Animal Hair.)

Hyaluronic Acid.
A protein found in umbilical cords and the fluids around the joints. Used as a cosmetic oil. Alternatives: plant oils.

Hydrocortisone.
(See Cortisone.)
Hydrolyzed Animal Protein.
In cosmetics, especially shampoo and hair treatments. Alternatives: soy protein, other vegetable proteins, amla oil (see alternatives to Keratin).

I
Imidazolidinyl Urea.
(See Urea.)

Insulin.
From hog pancreas. Used by millions of diabetics daily. Alternatives: synthetics, vegetarian diet and nutritional supplements, human insulin grown in a lab.

Isinglass.
A form of gelatin prepared from the internal membranes of fish bladders. Sometimes used in "clearing" wines and in foods. Alternatives: bentonite clay, "Japanese isinglass," agar-agar (see alternatives to Gelatin), mica, a mineral used in cosmetics.
Isopropyl Lanolate.
(See Lanolin.)

Isopropyl Myristate.
(See Myristic Acid.)

Isopropyl Palmitate.

Complex mixtures of isomers of stearic acid and palmitic acid. (See Stearic Acid).

K

Keratin.

Protein from the ground-up horns, hooves, feathers, quills, and hair of various animals. In hair rinses, shampoos, permanent wave solutions. Alternatives: almond oil, soy protein, amla oil (from the fruit of an Indian tree), human hair from salons. Rosemary and nettle give body and strand strength to hair.

L

Lactic Acid.

Found in blood and muscle tissue. Also in sour milk, beer, sauerkraut, pickles, and other food products made by bacterial fermentation. Used in skin fresheners, as a preservative, in the formation of plasticizers, etc. Alternative: plant milk sugars, synthetics.

Lactose.

Milk sugar from milk of mammals. In eye lotions, foods, tablets, cosmetics, baked goods, medicines. Alternatives: plant milk sugars.

Laneth.

(See Lanolin.)

Lanogene.

(See Lanolin.)

Lanolin. Lanolin Acids. Wool Fat. Wool Wax.
A product of the oil glands of sheep, extracted from their wool. Used as an emollient in many skin care products and cosmetics and in medicines. An allergen with no proven effectiveness. (See Wool for cruelty to sheep.) Derivatives: Aliphatic Alcohols, Cholesterin, Isopropyl Lanolate, Laneth, Lanogene, Lanolin Alcohols, Lanosterols, Sterols, Triterpene Alcohols. Alternatives: plant and vegetable oils.

Lanolin Alcohol.
(See Lanolin.)

Lanosterols.
(See Lanolin.)

Lard.
Fat from hog abdomens. In shaving creams, soaps, cosmetics. In baked goods, French fries, refried beans, and many other foods. Alternatives: pure vegetable fats or oils.

Leather. Suede. Calfskin. Sheepskin. Alligator Skin. Other Types of Skin.
Subsidizes the meat industry. Used to make wallets, handbags, furniture and car upholstery, shoes, etc. Alternatives: cotton, canvas, nylon, vinyl, ultrasuede, other synthetics.

Lecithin. Choline Bitartrate.

Waxy substance in nervous tissue of all living organisms. But, frequently obtained for commercial purposes from eggs and soybeans. Also from nerve tissue, blood, milk, corn. Choline bitartrate, the basic constituent of lecithin, is in many animal and plant tissues and prepared synthetically. Lecithin can be in eye creams, lipsticks, liquid powders, handcreams, lotions, soaps, shampoos, other cosmetics, and some medicines. Alternatives: soybean lecithin, synthetics.

Linoleic Acid.
An essential fatty acid. Used in cosmetics, vitamins. (See alternatives to Fatty Acids.)

Lipase.
Enzyme from the stomachs and tongue glands of calves, kids, and lambs. Used in cheese-making and in digestive aids. Alternatives: vegetable enzymes, castor beans.

Lipids.
(See Lipoids.)

Lipoids. Lipids.
Fat and fat-like substances that are found in animals and plants. Alternatives: vegetable oils.

M
Marine Oil.
From fish or marine mammals (including porpoises). Used in soap-making. Used as a

shortening (especially in some margarines), as a lubricant, and in paint. Alternatives: vegetable oils.

Methionine.
Essential amino acid found in various proteins (usually from egg albumen and casein). Used as a texturizer and for freshness in potato chips. Alternatives: synthetics.

Milk Protein.
Hydrolyzed milk protein. From the milk of cows. In cosmetics, shampoos, moisturizers, conditioners, etc. Alternatives: soy protein, other plant proteins.

Mink Oil.
From minks. In cosmetics, creams, etc. Alternatives: vegetable oils and emollients such as avocado oil, almond oil, and jojoba oil.

Monoglycerides. Glycerides. (See Glycerin.)
From animal fat. In margarines, cake mixes, candies, foods, etc. In cosmetics. Alternative: vegetable glycerides.

Musk (Oil).
Dried secretion painfully obtained from musk deer, beaver, muskrat, civet cat, and otter genitals. Wild cats are kept captive in cages in horrible conditions and are whipped around the genitals to produce the scent; beavers are trapped; deer are shot. In perfumes and in food flavorings. Alternatives: labdanum oil (which comes from various rockrose shrubs) and other

plants with a musky scent. Labdanum oil has no known toxicity.

Myristal Ether Sulfate.
(See Myristic Acid.)

Myristic Acid.
Organic acid in most animal and vegetable fats. In butter acids. Used in shampoos, creams, cosmetics. In food flavorings. Derivatives: Isopropyl Myristate, Myristal Ether Sulfate, Myristyls, Oleyl Myristate. Alternatives: nut butters, oil of lovage, coconut oil, extract from seed kernels of nutmeg, etc.

Myristyls.
(See Myristic Acid.)

N
"Natural Sources."
Can mean animal or vegetable sources. Most often in the health food industry, especially in the cosmetics area, it means animal sources, such as animal elastin, glands, fat, protein, and oil. Alternatives: plant sources.

Nucleic Acids.
In the nucleus of all living cells. Used in cosmetics, shampoos, conditioners, etc. Also in vitamins, supplements. Alternatives: plant sources.

O

Ocenol.
(See Oleyl Alcohol.)

Octyl Dodecanol.
Mixture of solid waxy alcohols. Primarily from stearyl alcohol. (See Stearyl Alcohol.)

Oleic Acid.
Obtained from various animal and vegetable fats and oils. Usually obtained commercially from inedible tallow. (See Tallow.) In foods, soft soap, bar soap, permanent wave solutions, creams, nail polish, lipsticks, many other skin preparations. Derivatives: Oleyl Oleate, Oleyl Stearate. Alternatives: coconut oil. (See alternatives to Animal Fats and Oils.)

Oils.
(See alternatives to Animal Fats and Oils.)

Oleths.
(See Oleyl Alcohol.)

Oleyl Alcohol. Ocenol.
Found in fish oils. Used in the manufacture of detergents, as a plasticizer for softening fabrics, and as a carrier for medications. Derivatives: Oleths, Oleyl Arachidate, Oleyl Imidazoline.

Oleyl Arachidate.
(See Oleyl Alcohol.)

Oleyl Imidazoline.
(See Oleyl Alcohol.)

Oleyl Myristate.
(See Myristic Acid.)

Oleyl Oleate.
(See Oleic Acid.)

Oleyl Stearate.
(See Oleic Acid.)

P

Palmitamide.
(See Palmitic Acid.)

Palmitamine.
(See Palmitic Acid.)

Palmitate.
(See Palmitic Acid.)

Palmitic Acid.
From fats, oils (see Fatty Acids). Mixed with stearic acid. Found in many animal fats and plant oils. In shampoos, shaving soaps, creams. Derivatives: Palmitate, Palmitamine, Palmitamide. Alternatives: palm oil, vegetable sources.

Panthenol. Dexpanthenol. Vitamin B-Complex Factor. Provitamin B-5.
Can come from animal or plant sources or synthetics. In shampoos, supplements,

emollients, etc. In foods. Derivative: Panthenyl. Alternatives: synthetics, plants.

Panthenyl.
(See Panthenol.)

Pepsin.
In hogs' stomachs. A clotting agent. In some cheeses and vitamins. Same uses and alternatives as Rennet.

Placenta. Placenta Polypeptides Protein. Afterbirth.
Contains waste matter eliminated by the fetus. Derived from the uterus of slaughtered animals. Animal placenta is widely used in skin creams, shampoos, masks, etc. Alternatives: kelp. (See alternatives for Animal Fats and Oils.)

Polyglycerol.
(See Glycerin.)

Polypeptides.
From animal protein. Used in cosmetics. Alternatives: plant proteins and enzymes.

Polysorbates.
Derivatives of fatty acids. In cosmetics, foods.

Pristane.
Obtained from the liver oil of sharks and from whale ambergris. (See Squalene, Ambergris.) Used as a lubricant and anti-corrosive agent. In cosmetics. Alternatives: plant oils, synthetics.

Progesterone.
A steroid hormone used in anti-wrinkle face creams. Can have adverse systemic effects. Alternatives: synthetics.

Propolis.
Tree sap gathered by bees and used as a sealant in beehives. In toothpaste, shampoo, deodorant, supplements, etc. Alternatives: tree sap, synthetics.

Provitamin A.
(See Carotene.)

Provitamin B-5.
(See Panthenol.)

Provitamin D-2.
(See Vitamin D.)

R

Rennet. Rennin.
Enzyme from calves' stomachs. Used in cheese-making, rennet custard (junket), and in many coagulated dairy products. Alternatives: microbial coagulating agents, bacteria culture, lemon juice, or vegetable rennet.

Rennin.
(See Rennet.)

Resinous Glaze.
(See Shellac.)

Ribonucleic Acid.
(See RNA.)

RNA. Ribonucleic Acid.
RNA is in all living cells. Used in many protein shampoos and cosmetics. Alternatives: plant cells.

Royal Jelly.
Secretion from the throat glands of the honeybee workers that is fed to the larvae in a colony and to all queen larvae. No proven value in cosmetics preparations. Alternatives: aloe vera, comfrey, other plant derivatives.

S

Sable Brushes.
From the fur of sables (weasel-like mammals). Used to make eye makeup, lipstick, and artists' brushes. Alternatives: synthetic fibers.

Sea Turtle Oil.
(See Turtle Oil.)

Shark Liver Oil.
Used in lubricating creams and lotions. Derivatives: Squalane, Squalene. Alternatives: vegetable oils.

Sheepskin.
(See Leather.)

Shellac. Resinous Glaze.

Resinous excretion of certain insects. Used as a candy glaze, in hair lacquer, and on jewelry. Alternatives: plant waxes.

Silk. Silk Powder.
Silk is the shiny fiber made by silkworms to form their cocoons. Worms are boiled in their cocoons to get the silk. Used in cloth. In silk-screening (other fine cloth can be and is used instead). Taffeta can be made from silk or nylon. Silk powder is obtained from the secretion of the silkworm. It is used as a coloring agent in face powders, soaps, etc. Can cause severe allergic skin reactions and systemic reactions (if inhaled or ingested). Alternatives: milkweed seed-pod fibers, nylon, silk-cotton tree and ceiba tree filaments (kapok), rayon, and synthetic silks.

Snails.
In some cosmetics (crushed).

Sodium Caseinate.
(See Casein.)

Sodium Steroyl Lactylate.
(See Lactic Acid.)

Sodium Tallowate.
(See Tallow.)

Spermaceti. Cetyl Palmitate. Sperm Oil.
Waxy oil derived from the sperm whale's head or from dolphins. In many margarines. In skin creams, ointments, shampoos, candles, etc.

Used in the leather industry. May become rancid and cause irritations. Alternatives: synthetic spermaceti, jojoba oil, and other vegetable emollients.

Sponge (Luna and Sea).
A plant-like animal. Lives in the sea. Becoming scarce. Alternatives: synthetic sponges, loofahs (plants used as sponges).

Squalane.
(See Shark Liver Oil.)
Squalene.
Oil from shark livers, etc. In cosmetics, moisturizers, hair dyes, surface-active agents. Alternatives: vegetable emollients such as olive oil, wheat germ oil, rice bran oil, etc.

Stearamide.
(See Stearic Acid.)

Stearamine.
(See Stearic Acid.)

Stearamine Oxide.
(See Stearyl Alcohol.)

Stearates.
(See Stearic Acid.)

Stearic Acid.
Fat from cows and sheep and from dogs and cats euthanized in animal shelters, etc. Most often refers to a fatty substance taken from the stomachs of pigs. Can be harsh, irritating. Used

in cosmetics, soaps, lubricants, candles, hairspray, conditioners, deodorants, creams, chewing gum, food flavoring. Derivatives: Stearamide, Stearamine, Stearates, Stearic Hydrazide, Stearone, Stearoxytrimethylsilane, Stearoyl Lactylic Acid, Stearyl Betaine, Stearyl Imidazoline. Alternatives: Stearic acid can be found in many vegetable fats, coconut.

Stearic Hydrazide.
(See Stearic Acid.)

Stearone.
(See Stearic Acid.)

Stearoxytrimethylsilane.
(See Stearic Acid.)

Stearoyl Lactylic Acid.
(See Stearic Acid.)

Stearyl Acetate.
(See Stearyl Alcohol.)

Stearyl Alcohol. Sterols.
A mixture of solid alcohols. Can be prepared from sperm whale oil. In medicines, creams, rinses, shampoos, etc. Derivatives: Stearamine Oxide, Stearyl Acetate, Stearyl Caprylate, Stearyl Citrate, Stearyldimethyl Amine, Stearyl Glycyrrhetinate, Stearyl Heptanoate, Stearyl Octanoate, Stearyl Stearate. Alternatives: plant sources, vegetable stearic acid.

Stearyl Betaine.

(See Stearic Acid.)
Stearyl Caprylate.
(See Stearyl Alcohol.)

Stearyl Citrate.
(See Stearyl Alcohol.)

Stearyldimethyl Amine.
(See Stearyl Alcohol.)

Stearyl Glycyrrhetinate.
(See Stearyl Alcohol.)

Stearyl Heptanoate.
(See Stearyl Alcohol.)

Stearyl Imidazoline.
(See Stearic Acid.)

Stearyl Octanoate.
(See Stearyl Alcohol.)

Stearyl Stearate.
(See Stearyl Alcohol.)

Steroids. Sterols.
From various animal glands or from plant tissues. Steroids include sterols. Sterols are alcohol from animals or plants (e.g., cholesterol). Used in hormone preparation. In creams, lotions, hair conditioners, fragrances, etc. Alternatives: plant tissues, synthetics.

Sterols.
(See Stearyl Alcohol and Steroids.)

Suede. (See Leather.)

T

Tallow. Tallow Fatty Alcohol. Stearic Acid. Rendered beef fat. May cause eczema and blackheads. In wax paper, crayons, margarines, paints, rubber, lubricants, etc. In candles, soaps, lipsticks, shaving creams, other cosmetics. Chemicals (e.g., PCB) can be in animal tallow. Derivatives: Sodium Tallowate, Tallow Acid, Tallow Amide, Tallow Amine, Talloweth-6, Tallow Glycerides, Tallow Imidazoline. Alternatives: vegetable tallow, Japan tallow, paraffin and/or ceresin (see alternatives for Beeswax for all three). Paraffin is usually from petroleum, wood, coal, or shale oil.

Tallow Acid.
(See Tallow.)

Tallow Amide.
(See Tallow.)

Tallow Amine.
(See Tallow.)

Talloweth-6.
(See Tallow.)

Tallow Glycerides.
(See Tallow.)

Tallow Imidazoline.

(See Tallow.)

Triterpene Alcohols.
(See Lanolin.)

Turtle Oil. Sea Turtle Oil.
From the muscles and genitals of giant sea turtles. In soap, skin creams, nail creams, other cosmetics. Alternatives: vegetable emollients (see alternatives to Animal Fats and Oils).
Tyrosine.
Amino acid hydrolyzed from casein. Used in cosmetics and creams. Derivative: Glucose Tyrosinase.

U
Urea. Carbamide.
Excreted from urine and other bodily fluids. In deodorants, ammoniated dentrifices, mouthwashes, hair colorings, hand creams, lotions, shampoos, etc. Used to "brown" baked goods, such as pretzels. Derivatives: Imidazolidinyl Urea, Uric Acid. Alternatives: synthetics.

Uric Acid.
(See Urea.)

V
Vitamin A.

Can come from fish liver oil (e.g., shark liver oil), egg yolk, butter, lemongrass, wheat germ oil, carotene in carrots, and synthetics. It is an aliphatic alcohol. In cosmetics, creams, perfumes, hair dyes, etc. In vitamins, supplements. Alternatives: carrots, other vegetables, synthetics.

Vitamin B-Complex Factor.
(See Panthenol.)

Vitamin B Factor.
(See Biotin.)

Vitamin B-12.
Usually animal source. Some vegetarian B-12 vitamins are in a stomach base. Alternatives: some vegetarian B-12-fortified yeasts and analogs available. Plant algae discovered containing B-12, now in supplement form (spirulina). Also, B-12 is normally produced in a healthy body.

Vitamin D. Ergocalciferol. Vitamin D-2. Ergosterol. Provitamin D-2. Calciferol. Vitamin D-3.
Vitamin D can come from fish liver oil, milk, egg yolk, etc. Vitamin D-2 can come from animal fats or plant sterols. Vitamins D-2 and D-3 may be from fish oil. All the D vitamins can be in creams, lotions, other cosmetics, vitamin tablets, etc. Alternatives: plant and mineral sources, synthetics, completely vegetarian vitamins, exposure of skin to sunshine. Many other vitamins can come from animal sources.

Examples: choline, biotin, inositol, riboflavin, etc.

Vitamin H.
(See Biotin.)

W

Wax.
Glossy, hard substance that is soft when hot. From animals and plants. In lipsticks, depilatories, hair straighteners. Alternatives: vegetable waxes.

Whey.
A serum from milk. Usually in cakes, cookies, candies, and breads. In cheese-making. Alternatives: soybean whey.

Wool.
From sheep. Used in clothing. Ram lambs and old "wool" sheep are slaughtered for their meat. Sheep are transported without food or water, in extreme heat and cold. Legs are broken, eyes injured, etc. Sheep are bred to be unnaturally woolly, also unnaturally wrinkly, which causes them to get insect infestations around the tail areas. The farmer's solution to this is the painful cutting away of the flesh around the tail (called mulesing). "Inferior" sheep are killed. When shearing the sheep, they are pinned down violently and sheared roughly. Their skin is cut up. Every year, hundreds of thousands of shorn sheep die from exposure to cold. Natural

predators of sheep (wolves, coyotes, eagles, etc.) are poisoned, trapped, and shot. In the U.S., overgrazing of cattle and sheep is turning more than 150 million acres of land to desert. "Natural" wool production uses enormous amounts of resources and energy (to breed, raise, feed, shear, transport, slaughter, etc., the sheep). Derivatives: Lanolin, Wool Wax, Wool Fat. Alternatives: cotton, cotton flannel, synthetic fibers, ramie, etc.

Wool Fat.
(See Lanolin.)

Wool Wax.
(See Lanolin.)

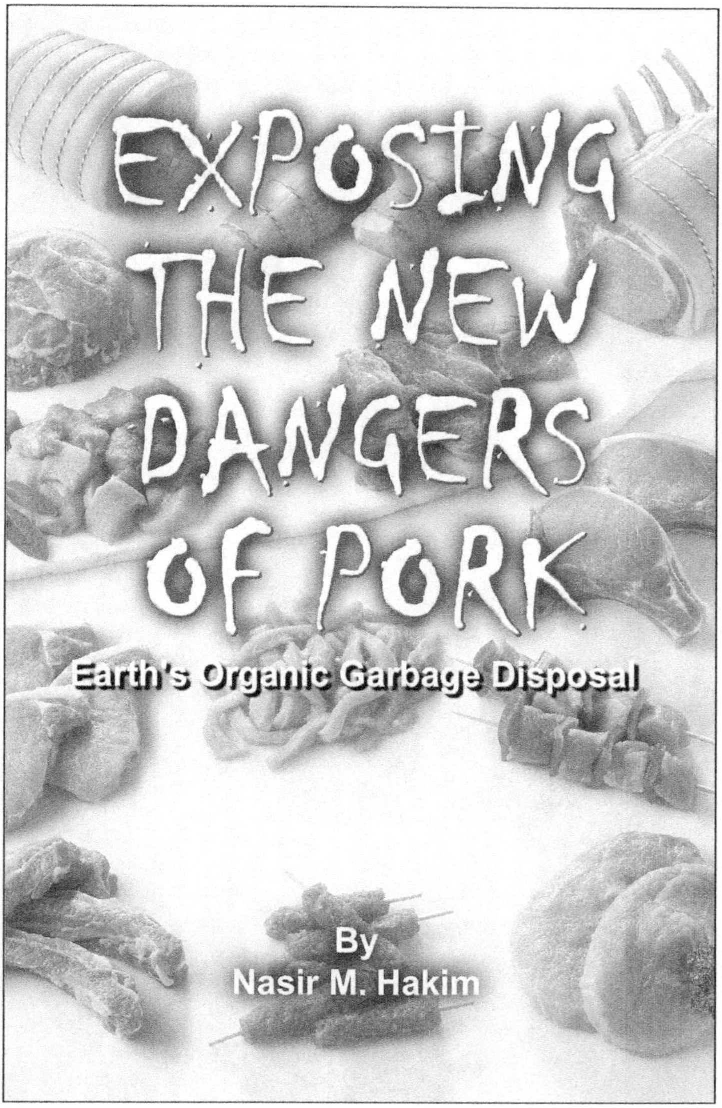

For more information Call **602 466-7347**
or visit:
www.memps.com
See Back cover for contact information.

Made in the USA
Monee, IL
13 September 2026

62975584R00164